THE HERBAL BATH & BODY BOOK

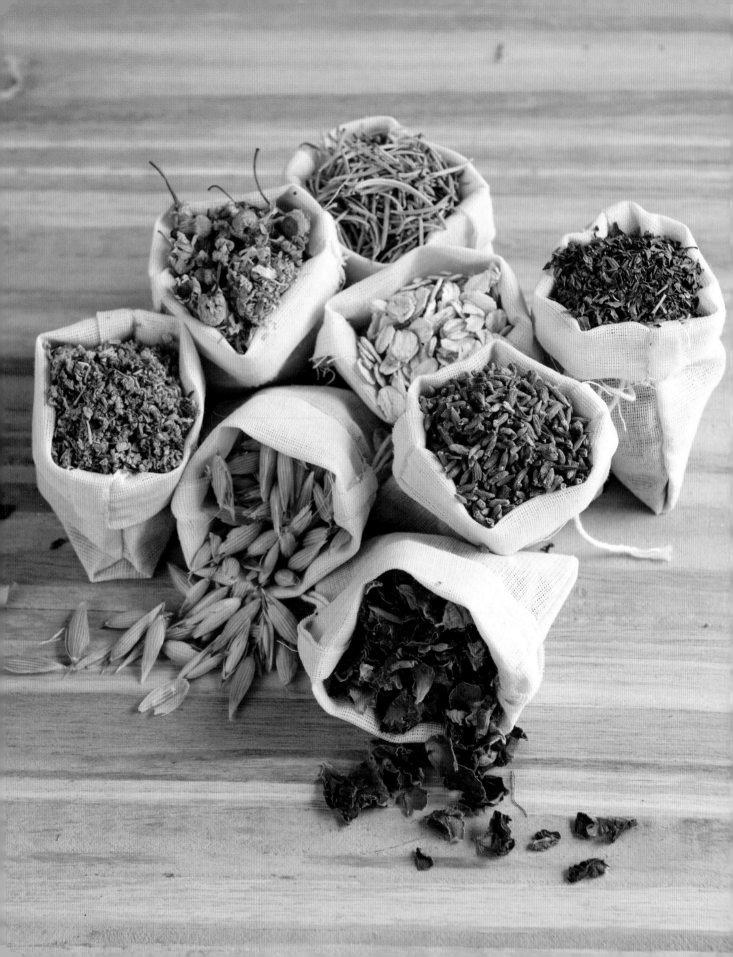

THE HERBAL BATH & BODY BOOK

Create Custom Natural Products for Hair and Skin

Heather Lee Houdek

 LARK

LARK

An Imprint of Sterling Publishing
387 Park Avenue South
New York, NY 10016

ISBN 978-1-4547-0849-0

Library of Congress Cataloging-in-Publication Data

Houdek, Heather Lee.
  The herbal bath & body book / Heather Lee Houdek.
    pages cm
  Includes index.
  ISBN 978-1-4547-0849-0
  1. Herbal cosmetics. 2. Beauty, Personal. 3. Baths--
Health aspects. I. Title. II. Title: Herbal bath and beauty
book.
  RA778.H79 2014
  646.7'2--dc23
                                        2013043171

Distributed in Canada by Sterling Publishing
c/o Canadian Manda Group, 165 Dufferin Street
Toronto, Ontario, Canada M6K 3H6
Distributed in the United Kingdom by GMC Distribution Services
Castle Place, 166 High Street, Lewes, East Sussex, England BN7 1XU
Distributed in Australia by Capricorn Link (Australia) Pty. Ltd.
P.O. Box 704, Windsor, NSW 2756, Australia

For information about custom editions, special sales, and premium and corporate purchases, please contact Sterling Special Sales at 800-805-5489 or specialsales@sterlingpublishing.com.

Email academic@larkbooks.com for information about desk and examination copies.
The complete policy can be found at larkcrafts.com.

Manufactured in China

2 4 6 8 10 9 7 5 3 1

larkcrafts.com

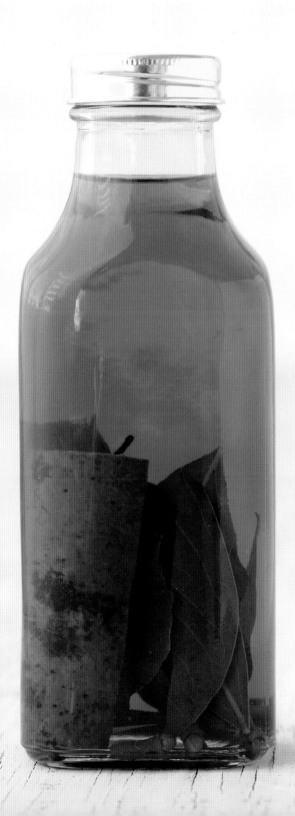

Welcome

I have always been a flora faerie. I've loved and felt a kinship with plants since I was a little girl. I fondly remember caring for my first houseplant—it hung in a basket in a sunny window in my bedroom for about 10 years.

My parents were hippies who raised me with a deep appreciation for the great outdoors. I learned about gardening and cultivars from my father, while my mother instilled in me a deep reverence for nature. This longtime love of plants logically led me to herbalism. I became interested in the subject when I was in college, where I began experimenting with natural medicine for the first time.

My interest in herbalism grew when I learned my mother had cancer. She fought a losing battle with the disease, during which I became disillusioned with the allopathic medicine system. This experience led to my full-on conversion to natural medicine, which I believe promotes health rather than sickness.

I studied holistic herbalism in school. During the journey that was my formal education, I learned the purposes of both the natural and allopathic medicine systems and how they can work together to promote the healing of the whole person. The experience of study changed my life forever, even as it returned me to my roots. It enabled me to reconnect with the healing power of the natural world and the plant friends that reside there. I learned that when I'm in balance with nature, the relationship provides me with both freedom and responsibility.

Making herbal medicines—especially body-care products—has become a special passion of mine. I love the do-it-yourself, hands-on approach. As an herbalism instructor, my favorite classes to teach are those on the making of herbal body products. My students are always so surprised to learn that they can easily reclaim this aspect of caring for themselves.

The idea that I could share my knowledge with a broader audience is what inspired me to write this book. Many people make the mistake of assuming that shampoos, salves, and lotions are too difficult and specialized to create at home. They think the skills and materials to make these products are beyond the reach of the layperson and confined to the special domain of corporations, chemists, and product developers. This is not the case!

I hope that this book will not only inspire and empower you to try the recipes for yourself, but also motivate you to pursue a deeper connection with plants. They are some of my greatest friends and allies. I've seen herbs do remarkable things. They've positively impacted my own health and life, as well as that of my friends.

It's in this spirit of healing that I offer you this book.

Heather

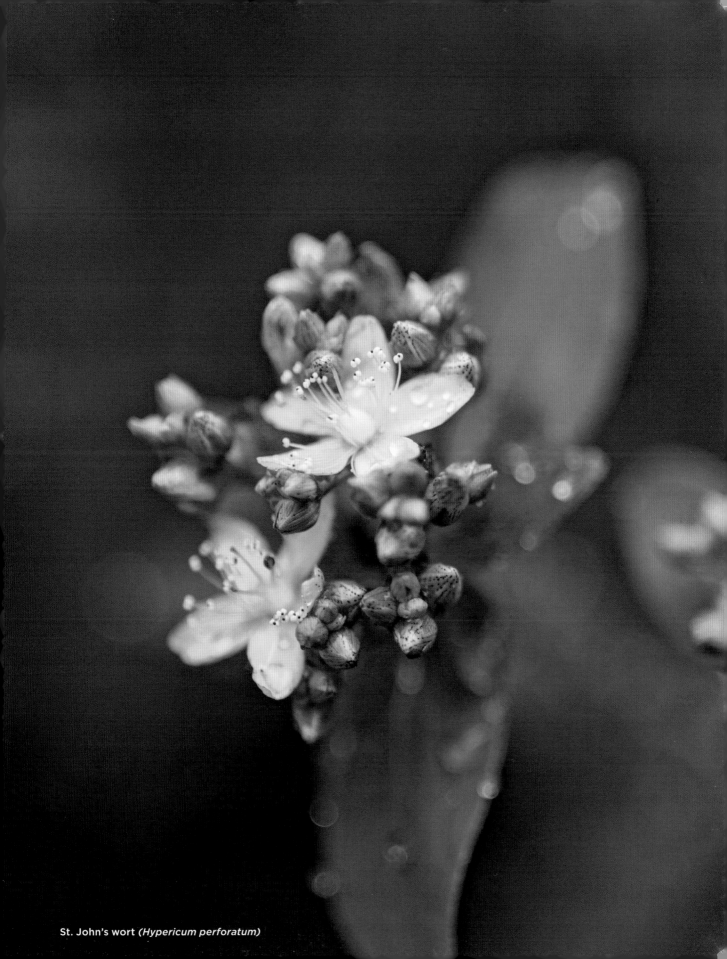

St. John's wort *(Hypericum perforatum)*

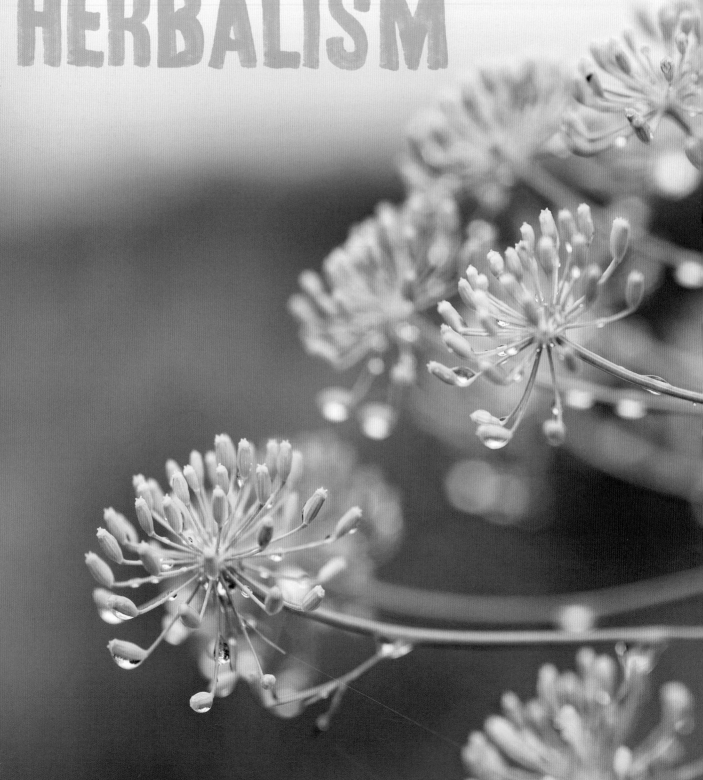

HERBS AND HERBALISM

WHAT IS HERBALISM?

Herbalism is the age-old practice of using plants and plant parts as medicine to maintain health and cure illness. No one knows for certain when plants were first employed as healing agents, but evidence suggests that humans turned to them for medicinal reasons thousands and thousands of years ago.

People's relationship with the natural world—particularly plants—predates recorded history. Ancient humans used plants for a variety of purposes—for food, fuel, and medicine. They wove plants into clothing, made them into decorations, and integrated them into special ceremonies. They used them to alter the mind and uplift the spirit. Our species evolved along with plants, but we often forget that without the symbiotic exchange of oxygen and carbon dioxide that takes place between us and our plant friends, neither of us would survive. Yet our relationship goes far beyond that exchange. Plants help us do more than merely survive—they allow us to thrive.

In as much as 75% of the world, herbalism is the main or only form of medicine available. Today, more and more consumers in the United States and Europe are turning to herbs as they fail to find relief in allopathic—or mainstream—medicine and struggle with the harsh side effects that often accompany prescription medications. All things considered, it's no surprise that an increasing number of people are seeking out natural alternatives and embracing age-old wellness practices.

Like many people, I once believed that herbs were harmless substances that could cure just about anything. But once I began studying them, I learned that—like any other medication—herbs have powerful side effects. In extreme cases, they can cause sickness or even death. Because they're powerful healing agents, herbs deserve respect, and you should approach them with the same caution you would any other medication. Consult a trained practitioner, herbalist, or naturopathic doctor before you use herbs internally. If you're taking a prescription drug, you should exercise extra caution because herbs can interact poorly with other medications.

Most herbalists take a holistic approach to healing. They view the human body as a unified whole rather than as an organism composed of separate systems. They consider an individual's mind, body, spirit, and history before assigning a protocol, which they monitor and, if necessary, tweak. If you suffer from a chronic illness, an herbalist will usually look for a root cause instead of simply treating your symptoms.

HERBS AREN'T JUST PLANTS!

We think of herbs as plants or plant parts that have medicinal qualities. However, in many medicine systems, especially those dating back to ancient times, plants weren't the only herbs. Any object could have sacred, healing properties. In many traditions, crystals, dirt, feathers, bones, rocks, and insects were considered herbs. I find this bit of ancient knowledge inspiring. Keep it in mind as you craft your own body-care products.

In my opinion, herbs work best as preventative medicine, although they can be used to address chronic and acute conditions. Because plants evolved along with humans, in many cases their healing properties are more easily assimilated into our bodies than chemicals that are isolated from natural products or those that are made through chemical synthesis. I've used herbs to treat everything from pink eye and the flu to thyroid problems and high blood pressure. Again, it's important to remember that herbs aren't miracle cures or magic pills. Using them as a treatment requires patience and dedication. People with acute conditions often take a number of herbs multiple times a day (as often as every 15 minutes), and the results don't happen overnight. Herbs should be taken for at least six weeks to treat chronic conditions or long-term problems, after which their effects can be assessed. This may seem like a long time, but once they manifest themselves, the benefits of herbs—radiant skin and a healthier body—are undeniable.

The same principles apply to the body-care recipes in this book. Don't expect your dandruff or wrinkles to disappear overnight when you start using them. Think long-term. Over time, the regular application of these products will lead to lasting and effective healing changes in your body.

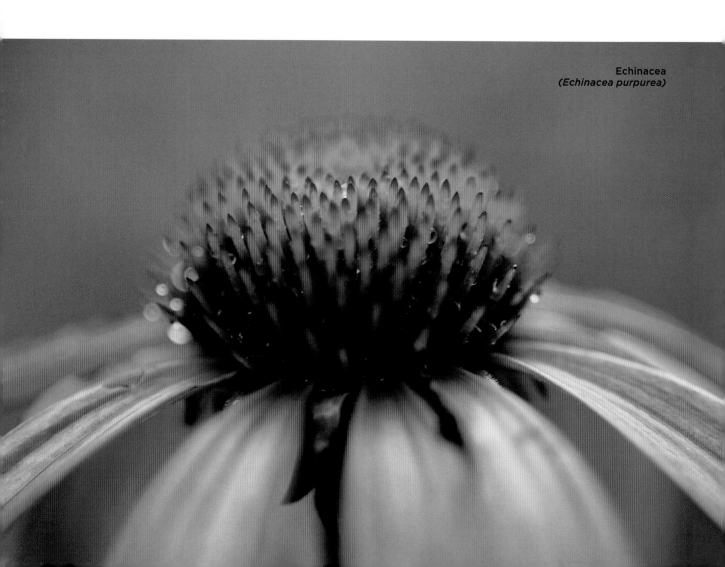

Echinacea
(Echinacea purpurea)

Most of the herbs listed on the following pages are easy to find. Many are simple to grow, too, if you have a garden or want to try them out in a pot on the windowsill. If you decide to grow your own, check out the great sources for herb seeds listed in the Additional Resources section on page 139.

If you choose to harvest your herbs from the "wild" (a process known as wild-crafting), consider the following practices:

Know Your Herbs

Make sure you know what you're harvesting. Buy one of the guidebooks listed in the Additional Resources section on page 138 and become familiar with it, or take a class in plant identification. Many herbs have lookalikes that are potentially toxic. Identifying plants correctly is VERY important. If you're in doubt, ask someone who knows, or bypass the plant altogether.

Harvest in a Safe Spot

You'll often see herbs growing by the side of the road, but you should never harvest them at a place where road runoff occurs. Roads are a source of toxic chemicals and heavy metals. Weeds growing near a road may contain both.

Drying Herbs

Most of the recipes in this book call for dried herbs. You can dry herbs in a number of different ways. If you have a dehydrator, then you're all set, although hanging bunches of herbs in a sunny window to dry the old-fashioned way is an equally effective method. You can also chop up the herbs, place them between two screens (such as pieces of window screens), and put them outside in the sun.
You'll be amazed at how quickly they'll dry!

Your body-care products will be no less amazing if you buy your herbs. You'll find listings for purchasing them in the Additional Resources section on page 139. I usually use a mixture of homegrown, wild-crafted, and purchased herbs to make my body-care products.

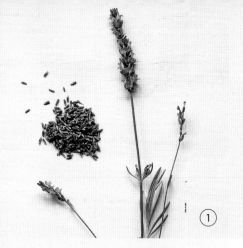

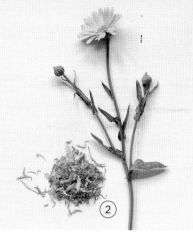

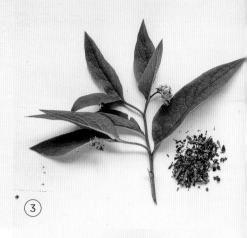

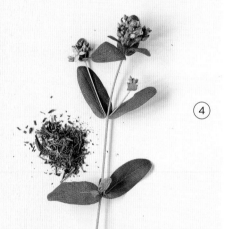

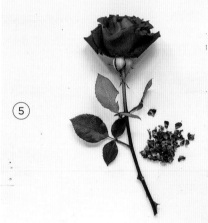

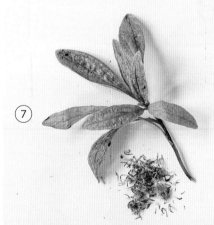

HERBS—MY TOP 20

In this chapter, I discuss some of my favorite herbs—the ones I use the most in my body-care products. My focus is on their external usage, although I do address some of their medical applications. For more information on how to use these and other herbs internally, check out the books listed in the Additional Resources section on page 138 or talk with a qualified practitioner.

The Importance of Latin Names

I've included a Latin and a common name for each herb. Herbalists use Latin names to avoid confusion over the identity of a plant. Many plants share common names, which can differ from place to place, but each plant has only one Latin name. Knowing it is a surefire way of identifying your specimen.

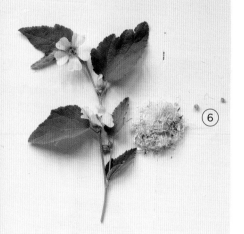

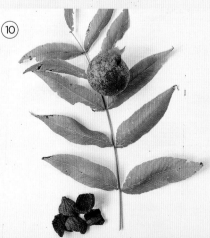

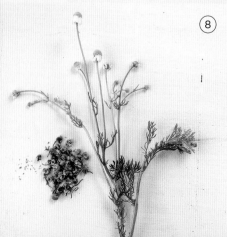

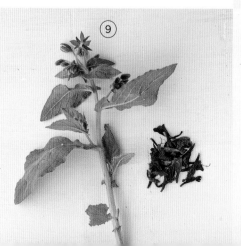

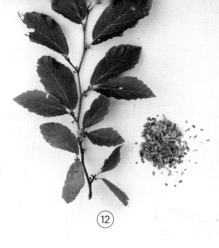

(11)

(12)

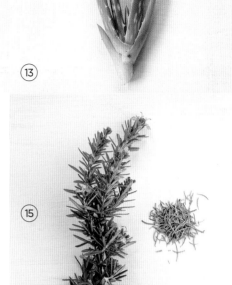

(13)

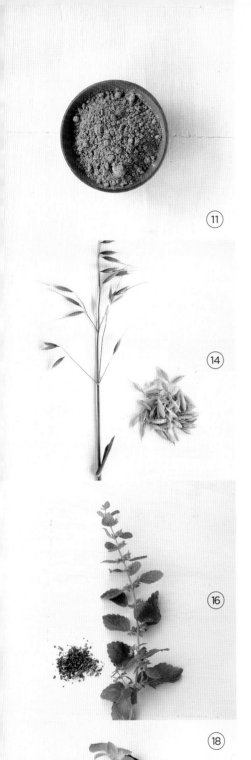

(14)

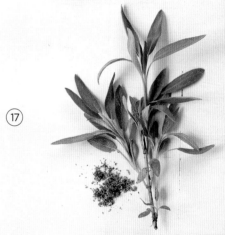

(15)

1. Lavender (Lavendula spp.)
2. Calendula
   (Calendula officinalis)
3. Comfrey (Symphytum officinale)
4. St. John's wort
   (Hypericum perforatum)
5. Rose (Rosa spp.)
6. Marshmallow plant
   (Althaea officinalis)
7. Arnica (Arnica montana)
8. Chamomile (Matricaria recutita)
9. Borage (Borago officinalis)
10. Black Walnut (Juglans nigra)
11. Henna (Lawsonia inermis)
12. Witch hazel
    (Hamamelis virginiana)
13. Aloe vera (Aloe vera)
14. Oats (Avena sativa)
15. Rosemary
    (Rosmarinus officinalis)
16. Lemon balm
    (Melissa officinalis)
17. Sage (Salvia officinalis)
18. Chickweed (Stellaria media)
19. Peppermint (Mentha piperita)
20. Nettle (Urtica dioica)

(16)

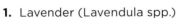

(17)

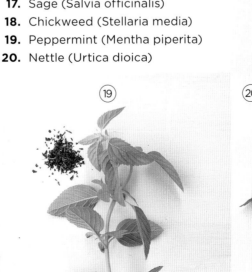

(18)

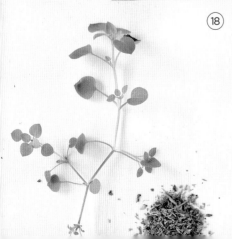

(19)

(20)

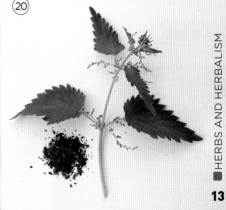

LAVENDER

(Lavendula spp.)

Celebrated as a beautifully scented and soothing herb, lavender is one of the best remedies for burns, stings, cuts, and irritated skin, thanks to its antibacterial properties. Also lauded for its sedative actions, it calms anxiety and tension.

Parts used: flowers

You're probably familiar with the delicate purple flowers and piney floral scent of lavender. A favorite in the garden—many people cultivate it—lavender is also used as a scent in cosmetics and perfumes. Remember the lavender sachets grandma put in her underwear drawer? She knew what she was doing! An all-around relaxer, the scent of lavender can soothe the nervous system, act as a mood booster, assist with insomnia, and ease headaches, especially those caused by stress.

The flowering tops of lavender plants can be put into cosmetic preparations, while lavender essential oil is in a class by itself. It's one of the few essential oils that can be used neat, which means it doesn't have to be diluted. You can apply it as is, directly to the skin. Lavender essential oil soothes the nerves, helps with headaches, and is excellent for all types of skin problems. It's especially helpful for sensitive skin that may be irritated by other essential oils.

I carry lavender essential oil in my purse for first-aid purposes. It's antimicrobial, which means it's great for killing germs in minor cuts, scrapes, bug bites, and burns. It also has anti-inflammatory, analgesic, and skin-regenerative properties that make it a wonderful treatment for acne-prone skin. I've found it especially useful in healing pimples and breakouts. The essential oil also has the amazing ability to be normalizing, which means that it stimulates while it relaxes. It can be especially useful after a stressful day at work, when you have frazzled nerves and need to relax but aren't necessarily ready for bed. The essential oil works wonders in muscle rubs and ointments that address pain.

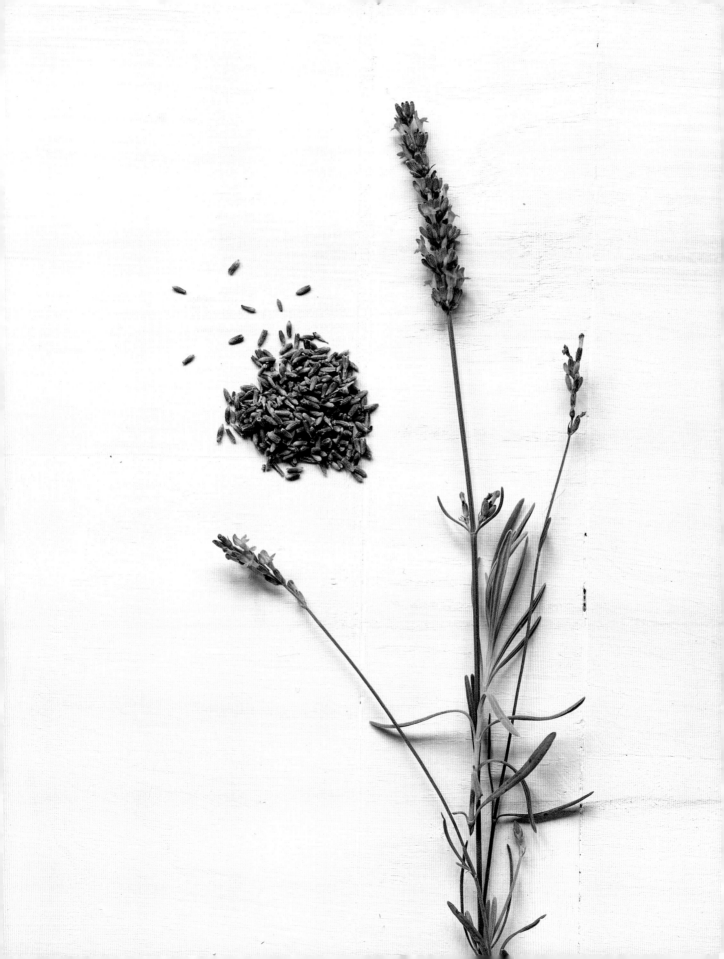

CALENDULA

(Calendula officinalis)

A good friend to skin, this cheerful yellow flower is one of the best options for treating inflammation and healing minor burns and bruises.

Parts used: flowers

Calendula is a cheery yellow flower that resembles the daisy. It's easy to grow in the garden and flowers at the height of summer. Calendula petals are used in many of the herbal preparations in this book. A powerful wound healer both internally and externally, calendula promotes rapid cell growth and acts as an antiseptic. It's used externally to treat bruises, burns, ulcers, and sores. It also reduces the inflammation and irritation that accompany acne. It makes a sunny herbal oil that's very healing to the skin.

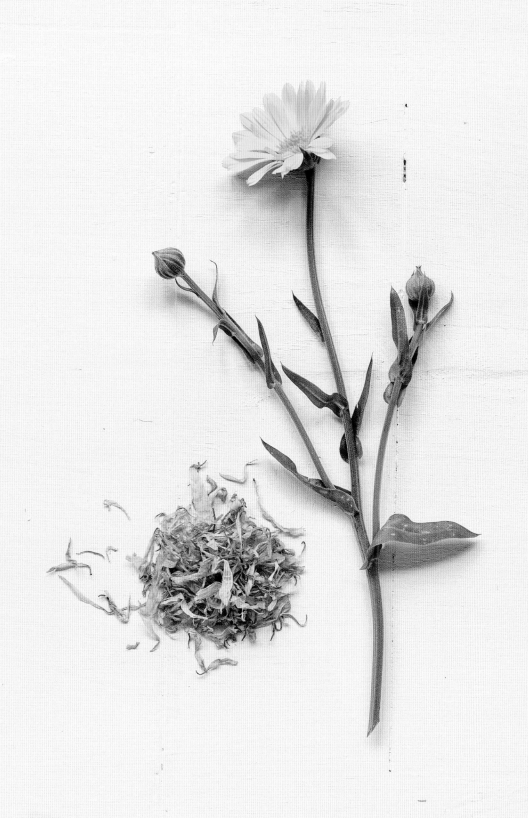

COMFREY

(Symphytum officinale)

This impressive wound healer works wonders in oils and salves to repair damage.

Parts used: root and leaves

Comfrey is a tough, hardy plant with big leaves and bell-shaped flowers that's very easy to grow. Herbalists use the root, rhizome, and leaf of the plant. The root and the leaf have similar properties, but the root is stronger. Comfrey is one of the best wound-healing herbs. It's excellent for treating torn ligaments, strains, bruises, and injuries to the bones and joints. It contains the constituent allantoin, which stimulates cell proliferation and augments wound healing both inside and out. Comfrey is so effective at forming new layers of tissue that care must be taken when it's applied to deep wounds. It can cause tissue to form over a wound before healing has taken place beneath the surface, which can lead to an abscess. Comfrey makes a wonderful greenish oil or salve for healing minor wounds. As a rub, it's good for treating deeper or internal wounds. Astringing and toning, it's useful for aging or weather-damaged skin and can help diminish scars and wrinkles.

Comfrey has been administered both internally and externally for hundreds of years. It's been used as a pregnancy tonic and as a treatment for cancer, but recent research suggests that it may be harmful to ingest. If you plan to take comfrey internally, do some research first and consult a trained practitioner.

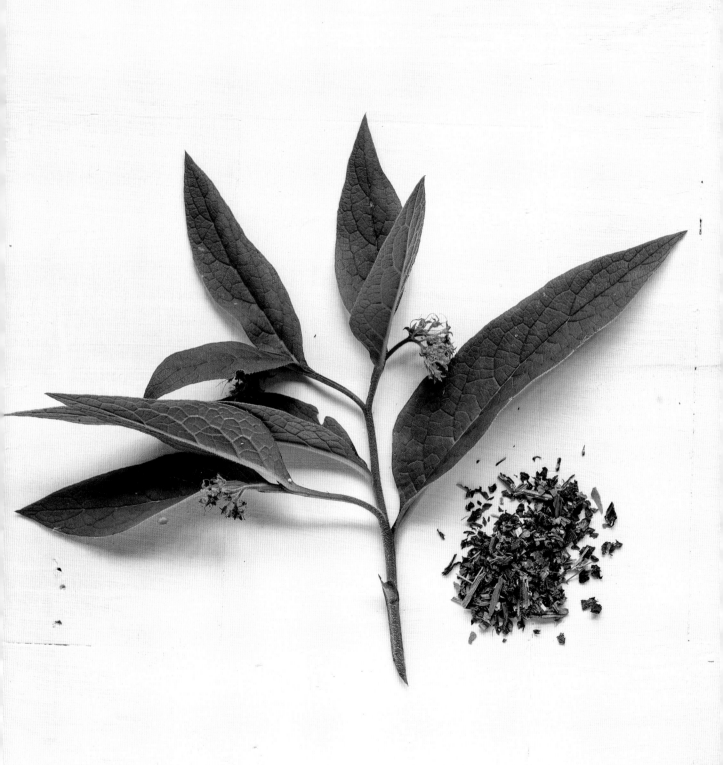

ST. JOHN'S WORT

(Hypericum perforatum)

Highly regarded in recent years for its effect on nervous tension and anxiety, St. John's wort is also a notable anti-inflammatory and healing agent for nerve damage and skin trauma.

Parts used: herb tops and flowers

St. John's wort is one of my favorite herbs! It blooms around the time of the summer solstice and is easy to identify thanks to the translucent oil glands in its leaves, which are unique to Hypericum perforatum. The glands appear as little dots when the leaves are held up to the light. The flowering tops of St. John's wort are used in herbal preparations.

St. John's wort has long been used in Europe (as a tincture, St. John's wort is very effective). It's a terrific aid for stress, anxiety, mild depression, chronic fatigue, personality disorders, and seasonal affective disorder (it's said to "bring the sun in"). In the dead of winter, there's nothing like putting on lotion made with St. John's wort oil that was infused during the height of summer. It has the uncanny ability to make you feel the warmth and abundance of that season. St. John's wort works well as a pain reliever because of the advantageous way it acts on the nervous system. It's used in treatments for the nerve damage that can occur with burns, neuralgia, and other skin trauma, and for infections such as herpes that have a nerve component. It has also been administered as a treatment for urinary tract and lung problems. St. John's wort is thought to cause photosensitivity, but the oil is actually very helpful for sunburns.

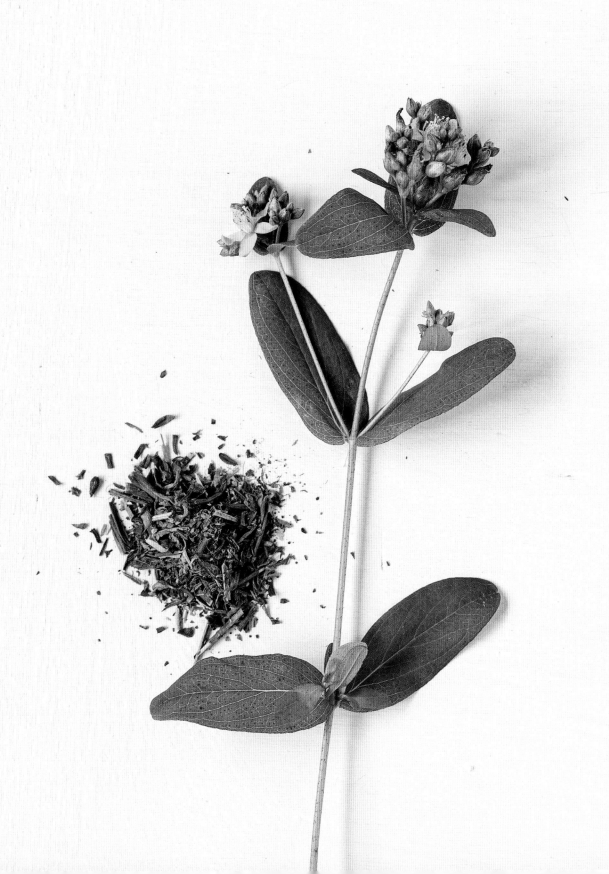

ROSE

(Rosa spp.)

While a rose is certainly a perfume-packed beauty, it's also a powerful astringent and mood lifter. It is soothing, cooling, and moisturizing.

Parts used: flowers

Everyone knows this classic flower and its heavenly scent. The rose is a powerful symbol of love, and that can be considered a form of medicine in itself! Who doesn't feel better after smelling a beautiful bouquet of roses? The unfurling petals of the flower seem to open our hearts.

But roses aren't merely to be admired in a vase or enjoyed on Valentine's Day. Rose petals are extremely useful in herbal skin-care products. They're astringent and toning, which means they're great for shrinking pores and maintaining healthy skin. Rose hips are the "fruit" of the rose plant. Bright red, with a shape that resem-bles a bulb or a berry, rose hips have more vitamin C than citrus fruits or other herbs. Instead of that glass of OJ you have in the morning, try rose-hip tea. It has a delightful pink color and a tart, fruity flavor.

The essential oil of the rose can be helpful with reducing wrinkles, lifting sagging skin, and bringing a youthful glow to the complexion. The astringent properties of rose are also wonderful for strengthening hair at the roots. When used in shampoos or rinses, rose can give hair a healthy shine. Additionally, the smell of roses has a relaxing effect. It can lift the spirit, act as an aphrodisiac, and—of course!—invoke romantic feelings.

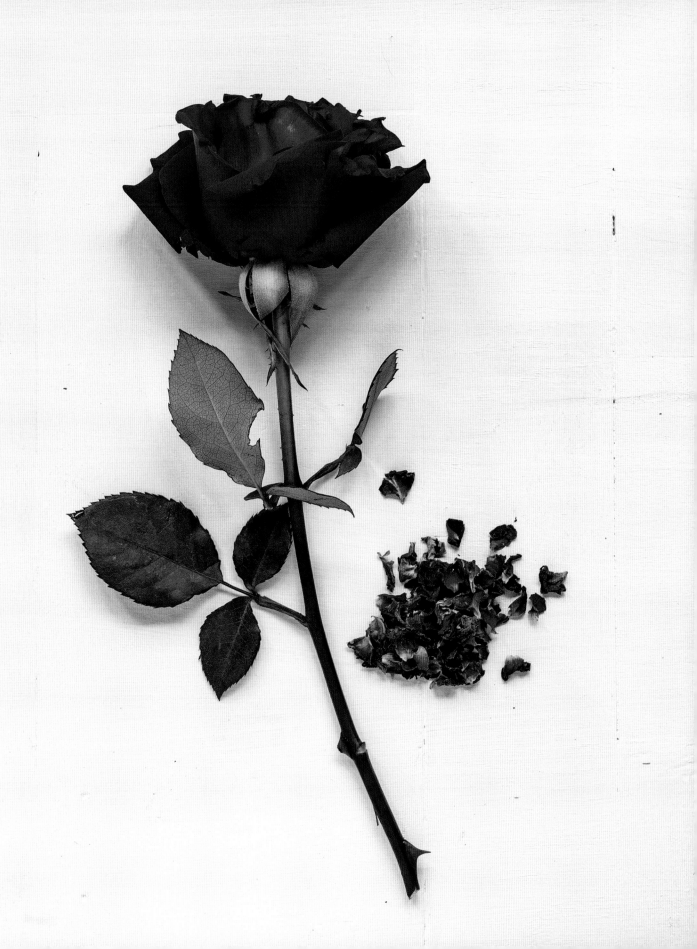

MARSHMALLOW PLANT

(Althaea officinalis)

This naturally high mucilage plant can really alleviate irritation caused by dryness.

Parts used: root and leaves

The marshmallow plant serves so many different purposes! Its leaves and flowers are useful as food. Its root—the most potent part of the plant—can be made into a tea for treating sore throats, diarrhea, constipation, and bronchial inflammation. (The ancient Egyptians made a honey-sweetened marshmallow preparation to relieve sore throats.) Confectioners in 19th-century France combined sap from the root with sugar, egg whites, and rosewater to make a sweet antecedent of the modern candy. Unlike their precursors, however, today's marshmallows don't contain any plant material.

Marshmallow root is also a wonderful skin healer that works well as a poultice. It's demulcent, meaning that it creates a soothing film on the skin that can help relieve minor pain and inflammation. In texture, it's mucilaginous—gooey and slippery—which is helpful for easing sensitive, irritated areas.

The root is especially useful for rosacea and for dry-skin conditions like psoriasis and eczema. It can even out the complexion, help with scarring, and soften and moisturize all skin types. It's great for aging skin, as it can help smooth fine lines and wrinkles.

Additionally, marshmallow root is useful in shampoos and hair rinses. It's a moisturizer that can improve dry, brittle hair. It can be used to repair weather-damaged or color-treated tresses, too. If you've got blonde or light-brown locks, be aware that marshmallow root may darken your hair slightly.

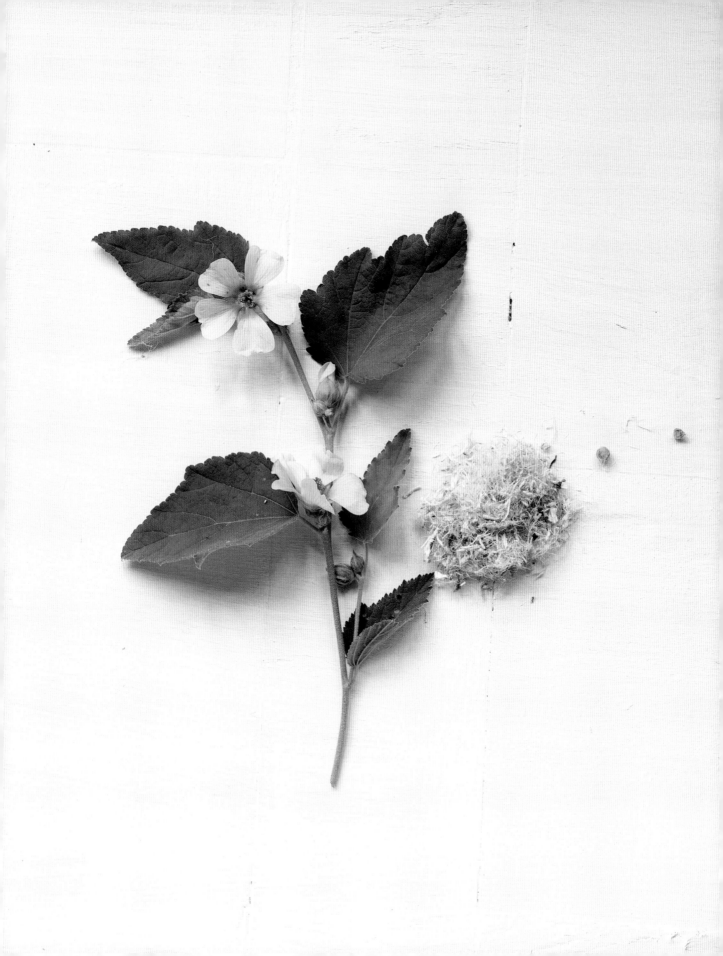

ARNICA

(Arnica montana)

Arnica is a reliable go-to for muscle aches, joint pain, sprains, and bruises as long as the skin is not broken.

Parts used: flowers

A plant that's native to Europe, arnica has been used medicinally since the 1500s. It grows in the western, mountainous regions of the United States. Often used in ointment and liniment preparations, arnica can soothe muscle aches and joint pain, reduce inflammation, and heal wounds. It's commonly used to ease sprains, swelling, and bruises. Years ago, after taking a bad tumble down some slippery stairs, I discovered the magic of arnica. My pain was greatly diminished by the arnica preparations I applied a few times a day, and my bruises healed relatively quickly.

Note: Arnica contains a toxin called helenalin that can be poisonous if ingested in large amounts. The plant itself can irritate the skin. It should never be applied to cuts, rashes, or open wounds. If ingested, the plant can cause dizziness, tremors, and heart irregularities. In large doses, it can cause vomiting and even death. Use arnica for external purposes only unless you're under the direct supervision of a trained medical practitioner. Homeopathic preparations of arnica are safe to ingest, though, and can be taken to treat sprains, bruises, overexertion, and even severe injuries.

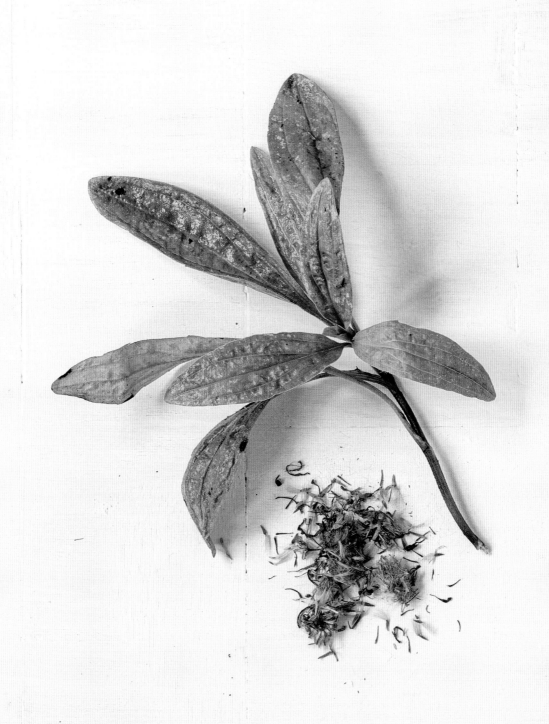

CHAMOMILE

(Matricaria recutita)

A favorite by many herbalists for its seemingly endless uses, chamomile is calming. This tension reliever is great for skin, body, and mind.

Parts used: flowers

Chamomile is a lovely little plant with tiny, daisy-like flowers. It's a common ingredient in bedtime and relaxation teas. It's also used for treating gastrointestinal upsets and for easing stress and anxiety. Because chamomile is gentle and safe, it's perfect to treat kids that are suffering from colic, nervous stress, infections, and stomach disorders! It's a great immune booster, too.

I use chamomile leaves and flowers in many of my body-care products. Chamomile contains the chemical constituents azulene and bisabolol. Both are powerful antioxidants that act as anti-inflammatory healing agents. Both can help prevent blemishes, stop the development of wrinkles, and improve skin pigmentation. Azulene is blue in color, and it gives the essential oil of chamomile its lovely blue hue.

In addition to treating dermatological diseases, aiding in relaxation, and soothing tense and aching muscles, chamomile works wonders when added to shampoo. It can bring out highlights and lighten hair.

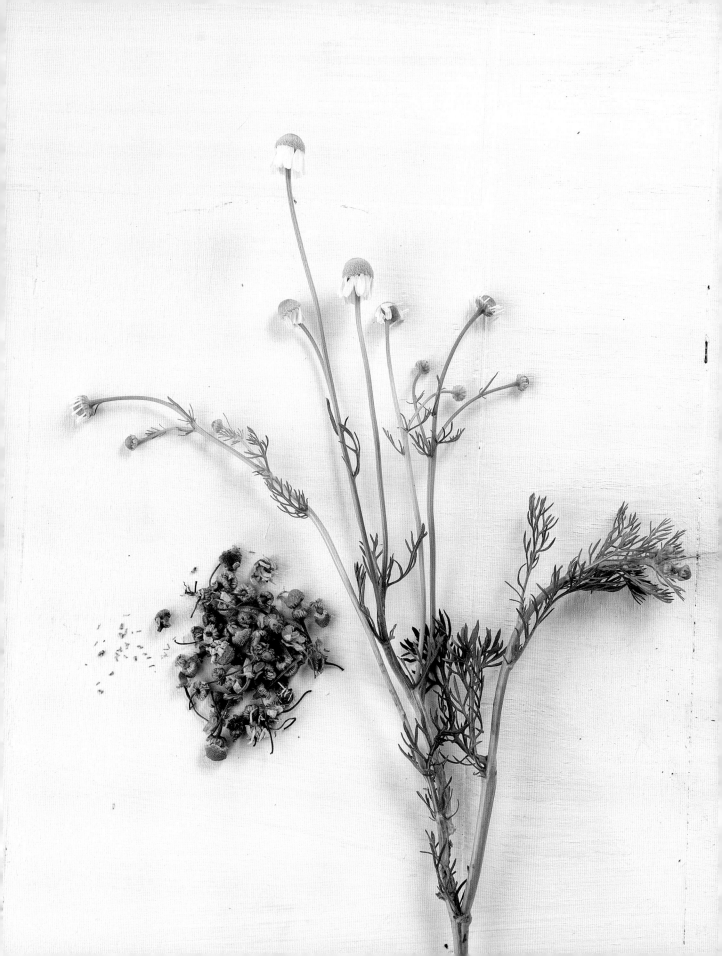

BORAGE

(Borago officinalis)

Commonly known as the "starflower," borage restores moisture and smoothness to dry and damaged skin, but can also provide relief to people who suffer from chronic skin disorders.

Parts used: leaves and flowers

Borage is another one of my favorite plants. With its star-shaped, purple flowers and fuzzy leaves, it reminds me of something from the fairy realm. Borage is native to southern Europe. It's a beautiful plant to have in the garden. Bees love it, and it helps them produce honey.

Mucilaginous in texture, borage is helpful for easing irritated or sensitive skin. It's especially beneficial as a wound healer and for treating acute skin eruptions and rashes. I love using borage in the bath. The dried flowers release a beautiful purple-blue color into the water. It makes for a lovely, relaxing soak that's healing to the skin.

As a medicinal herb, borage has a long history. It was traditionally used as a treatment for stress and anxiety. The ancient Romans favored it for the feelings of comfort and general uplift it provided. All over southern Europe, since ancient times, borage was viewed as a spirit booster and given as a remedy for depression, memory problems, and dizziness.

Borage is a diuretic herb. It's a helpful treatment for diseases of the urinary tract and for respiratory problems, fevers, ulcers, constipation, and the symptoms of menopause. A word of caution: Borage may contain harmful alkaloids, so you should use it internally with caution.

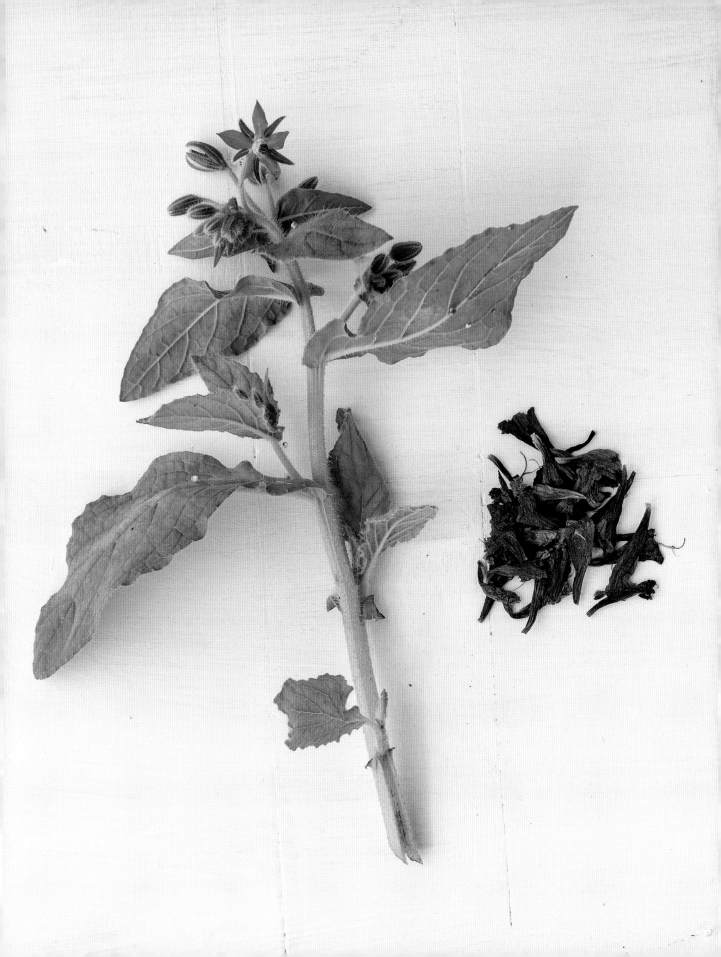

BLACK WALNUT

(Juglans nigra)

An antiviral and antifungal wonder, black walnut is fantastic in skin, hair, and scalp treatments.

Parts used: hulls

Black walnut trees are quite common. I have one growing in my yard, and I gather its green-hulled nuts in the autumn. Rich in high-quality oils and protein, the meat found in black walnuts is very nutritious and can be beneficial to people with wasting diseases.

If you're looking for something to treat skin issues, black walnut is antiparasitic and can clear up athlete's foot and other fungal infections, as well as infectious skin diseases. The hulls are useful in liniments, washes, and powders, but be warned: they will turn the skin a brownish-green color!

Black walnut hulls make a wonderful hair tonic and are a fabulous ingredient in shampoos and hair rinses. It's nutritious for the scalp and can help with dandruff, itchiness, and other scalp issues. It can be used to dye the hair and will darken it significantly. I've used black-walnut shampoo in the past, and many of my friends thought I'd colored my hair. The effect can be pretty dramatic.

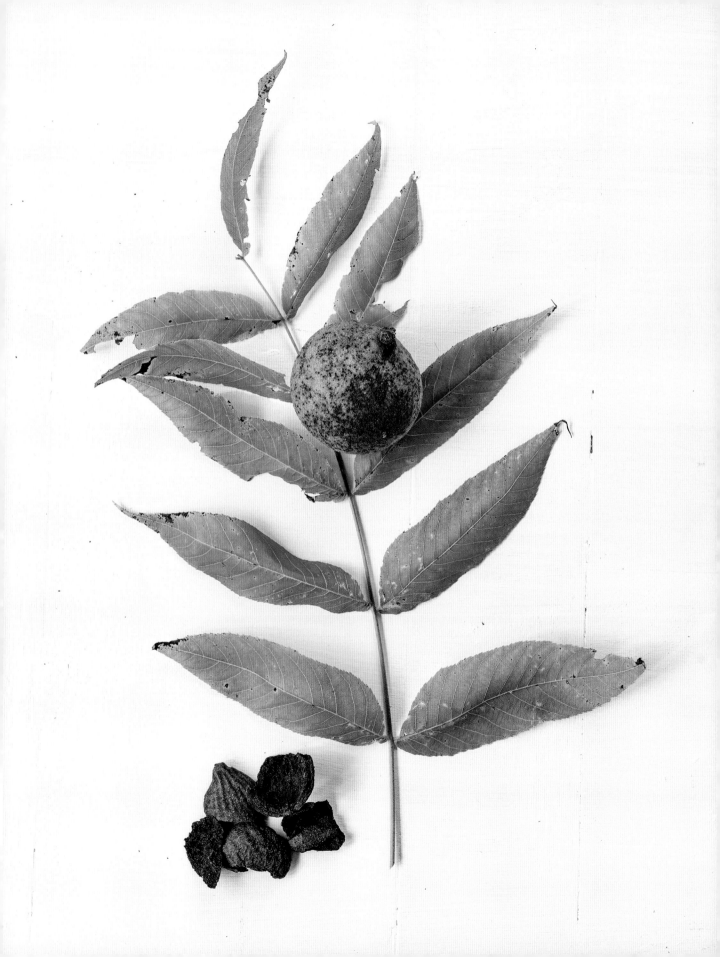

HENNA

(Lawsonia inermis)

Prized as a dye for hair, skin, and even fabrics, henna can come in a variety of colors. When used in the hair and scalp, it can have cooling and conditioning properties.

Parts used: leaves (dried and milled into a power)

Henna is also known as Egyptian privet. It has been used for at least 5,000 years as a medicine, talisman, ceremonial substance, and cosmetic for the hair and the body. The origins of the plant can be traced to North Africa and Asia. Henna is used to decorate the body in India and the Middle East. The henna-painting process is fun and magical. Once the henna is applied, it's allowed to dry and flake off. The first time I tried henna, I had a lotus painted on my arm. Because the design was very light, my initial reaction was, "That's it??" But after a few hours, the design got darker. By the next morning, it had turned a beautiful, rust-red color. Henna designs wear off naturally. They can last anywhere from a few days to a couple of weeks, depending on the number of times they're washed.

Today, henna serves mainly as a cosmetic colorant and a dye. A fun and completely natural way to color the hair, henna will give your tresses a red tone. (A word of warning: as a dye, it can be a bit messy to work with.) Henna is also an excellent conditioner that thickens and strengthens hair because it bonds to each individual hair shaft. Henna is astringent and tightens the scalp. It can help with dandruff, lice, and ringworm.

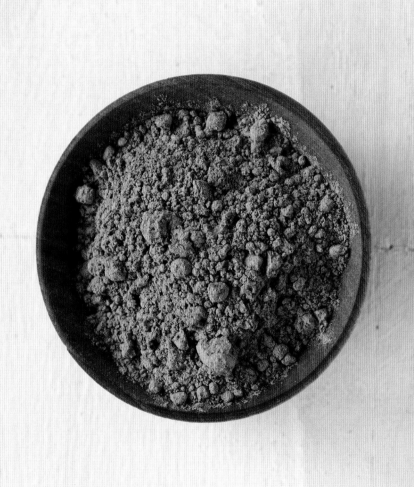

WITCH HAZEL

(Hamamelis virginiana)

Wonderfully astringent in nature, witch hazel can control surface bleeding, soothe and heal acne and oily skin, and tighten up and freshen the skin.

Parts used: leaves, bark, and twigs

This amazing little tree grows along streams and other areas where the soil is moist. I love the witch hazel because it's funky and seems to have a rebellious nature. The tree, which flowers in the winter, has asymmetrical leaves, crooked, angular branches, and wacky little yellow flowers with ridiculously long petals. Walking near the river by my house in early spring, I sometimes hear a crazy cracking noise—the sound of witch-hazel seeds popping open. What an incredible, unpredictable tree!

The extract from leaves, bark, and twigs of the tree can be used medicinally. Witch hazel is drying, cooling, sour, and very astringent. It can be used externally to stop bleeding and inflammation. It's analgesic (pain-relieving) and antibacterial, which makes it perfect for treating minor cuts and scrapes. It can also help with dermatitis, varicose veins, and broad-spectrum vein integrity.

Witch hazel is an antioxidant that's wonderful for the face. It shrinks pores, reduces the appearance of wrinkles, and firms sagging, aged skin. Thanks to its antibacterial properties, it's an excellent treatment for acne and for oily or problem skin.

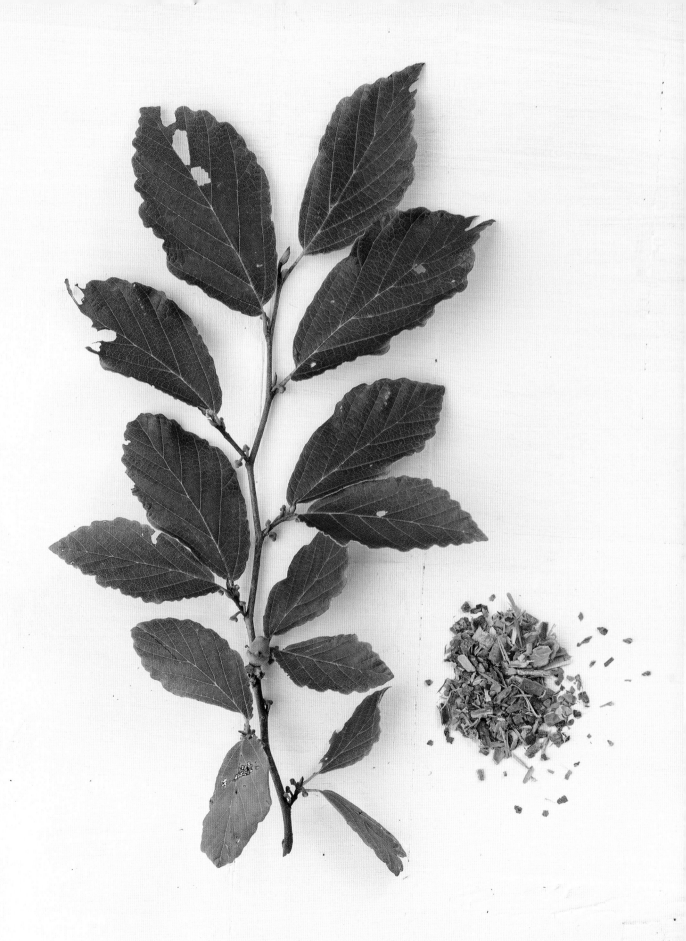

ALOE VERA

(Aloe vera)

Even as children we knew the value of aloe vera's cooling touch for burns, insect bites, and other skin irritations. But this plant is also a wonderful antiseptic and moisturizer.

Parts used: juice from leaves

Most of us are familiar with this friendly little houseplant. Aloe vera is first-aid in plant form! Its leaves can be used as a cooling emollient for skin abrasions, wounds, and burns (even radiation burns). Aloe vera gel has a pH of 4.3, making it an excellent ingredient for skin and hair preparations. A moisturizer that doesn't clog pores, it can calm and soothe sensitive skin. It's helpful for all sorts of dermatologic disorders, including pimples, acne, and rosacea.

Aloe vera contains aloin, a natural sunscreen that may block as much as 30% of the sun's rays. Not only is aloe vera great for treating sunburn, it can help prevent it in the first place.

Aloe-vera juice has been used for hundreds of years as a digestive aid and a laxative. People drink it today for a wide variety of reasons. It can boost the immune system and relieve symptoms associated with irritable bowel syndrome. But aloe vera (in any form) should be ingested with caution. In large doses, it can upset the stomach and cause cramping. Fresh aloe leaves should be peeled completely before they're used internally.

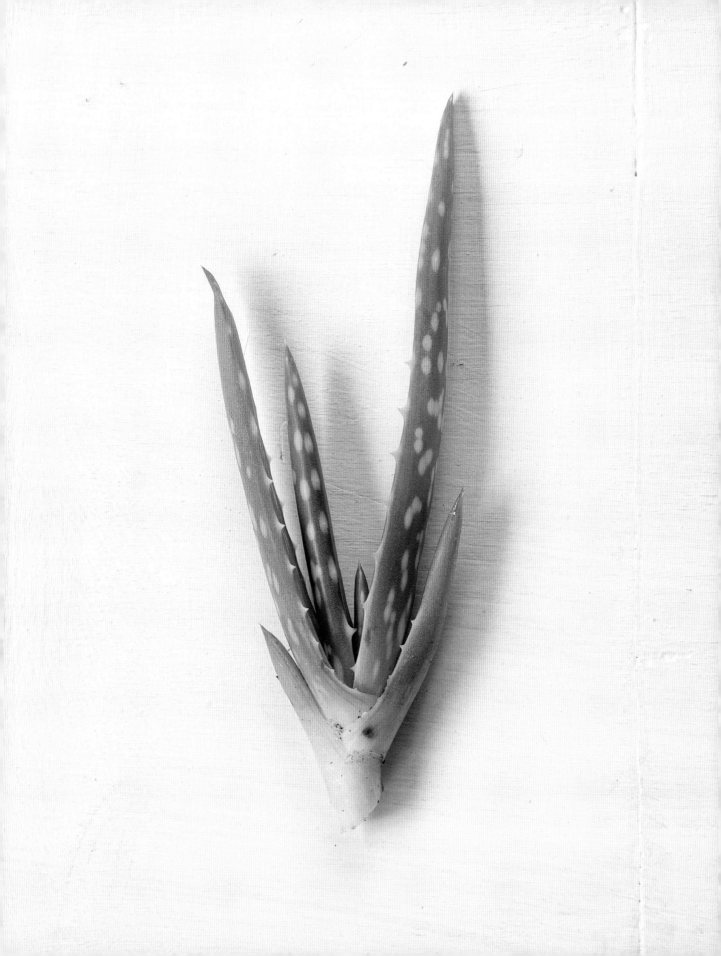

OATS

(Avena sativa)

This pantry staple doubles as an effective skin cleanser, exfoliate, moisturizer, and soother.

Parts used: seeds and whole plant

They're not just for breakfast! Oats are considered a key part of a heart-healthy diet. They're nutritious for the body, but did you know that they're also nourishing for the skin? The rolled oats in your kitchen have anti-inflammatory properties that help reduce spots, redness, and irritation. They're good for every type of complexion, including problem and sensitive skin. Oats are also helpful for soothing eczema, chicken pox, rashes, insect bites, and mild burns, including sunburns.

Because they contain a natural cleansing agent called saponin, oats are great for gently removing oil and dirt from the pores. Oats also have exfoliating properties.

Thanks to their somewhat gritty texture, they're perfect for removing dead skin cells and dry patches and smoothing fine lines and wrinkles. Oats are also emollient, which means that they hold and attract water and are thus naturally moisturizing. In general, oats seem to create a barrier of protection for the skin, keeping moisture in and environmental damage out.

Oats are not only soothing for the skin, they're soothing for the nerves! Rolled oats, milky oat tops, and oat straw are all amazing for the nervous system. They actually have the ability to rebuild the protective coating that surrounds the nerve cells, which can help to heal and restore balance to a frazzled nervous system.

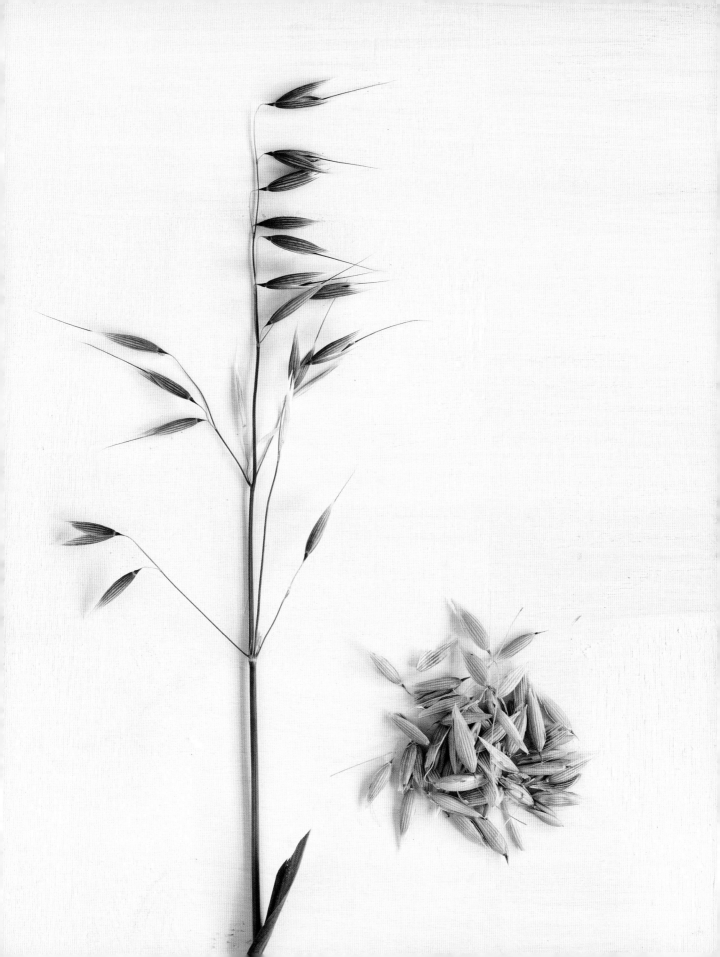

ROSEMARY

(Rosmarinus officinalis)

Rosemary has more to offer than just its stimulating scent. Helpful to aging, damaged, and oily complexions, it's also beneficial to the hair and scalp.

Parts used: leaves

Rosemary, an herb found in many kitchens, isn't just for cooking. Over the centuries, it's been used externally to treat everything from gout, muscular rheumatism, and sprains to tired or paralyzed limbs and nervous disorders.

I find that rosemary leaves are wonderful in body-care products. Rosemary is stimulating and rejuvenating for the skin, making it especially helpful for aging and damaged complexions. Its astringing qualities can help tone and tighten the skin and shrink pores. Rosemary also assists in stimulating blood flow to the skin, which can improve the complexion and aid in the reduction of lines and wrinkles. Rosemary's antimicrobial qualities make it a great treatment for acne and skin infections.

Rosemary is beneficial for hair, too. Traditionally, oil made with rosemary was used to treat and prevent baldness. The oil stimulates the hair follicles and facilitates blood flow to the scalp, which can encourage hair growth. Rosemary can help with itchy scalp and dandruff, and it's also good for oily hair. It can make any type of hair soft, shiny, and smooth. It can also bring out lowlights and darken hair.

Rosemary has long been known as a memory aid. The smell of rosemary and its essential oil is stimulating and revitalizing. "Rosemary for remembrance" is an old adage. When I was in herb school and needed a memory boost while studying, I spritzed myself with rosemary essential-oil spray. I like to use it in baths and body products as a pick-me-up either in the morning or after a long day. It can aid with exhaustion and help folks (like me!) who have a hard time waking up in the morning. A splash of rosemary astringent might be just what you need to start the day.

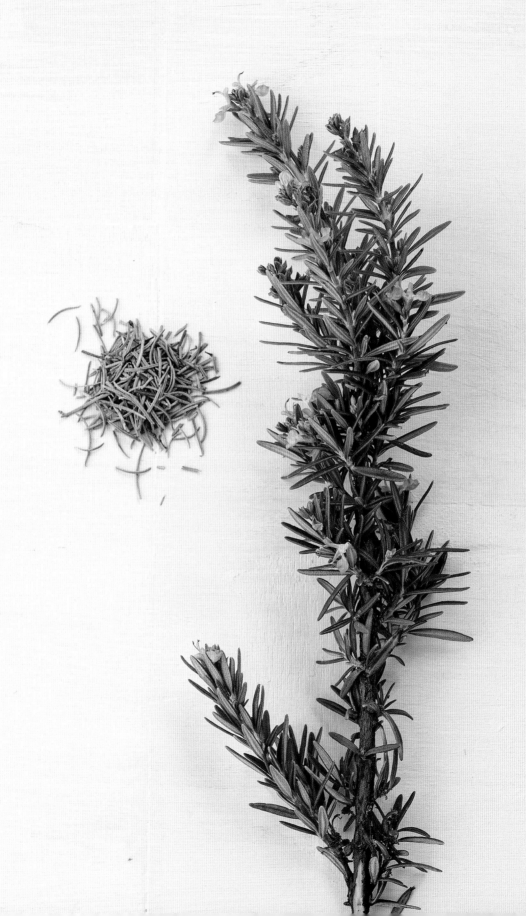

LEMON BALM

(Melissa officinalis)

Lemon balm is a delightful, mood-enhancing herb with a cheerful scent and powerful antiviral and antimicrobial properties that help with various skin infections.

Parts used: leaves

This delightful plant is incredibly easy to grow in the garden, but be careful—it likes to migrate and can take up residence in other parts of the garden or yard. If you decide to grow lemon balm, you should harvest the leaves.

Lemon balm is one of my favorite types of tea. It's especially refreshing in iced form in the summer. It's an effective antispasmodic for upset stomachs and helpful for bloating and gas. Try it with—and after—a meal!

Try using lemon balm as a mild sedative. It's a delicious remedy for insomnia, especially when the condition is caused by stress or anxiety. Lemon balm is also a mood booster. Its gladdening scent and invigorating essential oil are helpful for depression and nervous tension.

Lemon balm is known for its antimicrobial and antiviral properties. Both make it a very effective ingredient in salves for treating skin infections. Lemon balm is even helpful for herpes outbreaks and infected sores. Because it's anti-inflammatory and has cleansing properties that work to clear pores, it can help get rid of acne and prevent future breakouts. Lemon balm is especially good for acne in combination with oily skin.

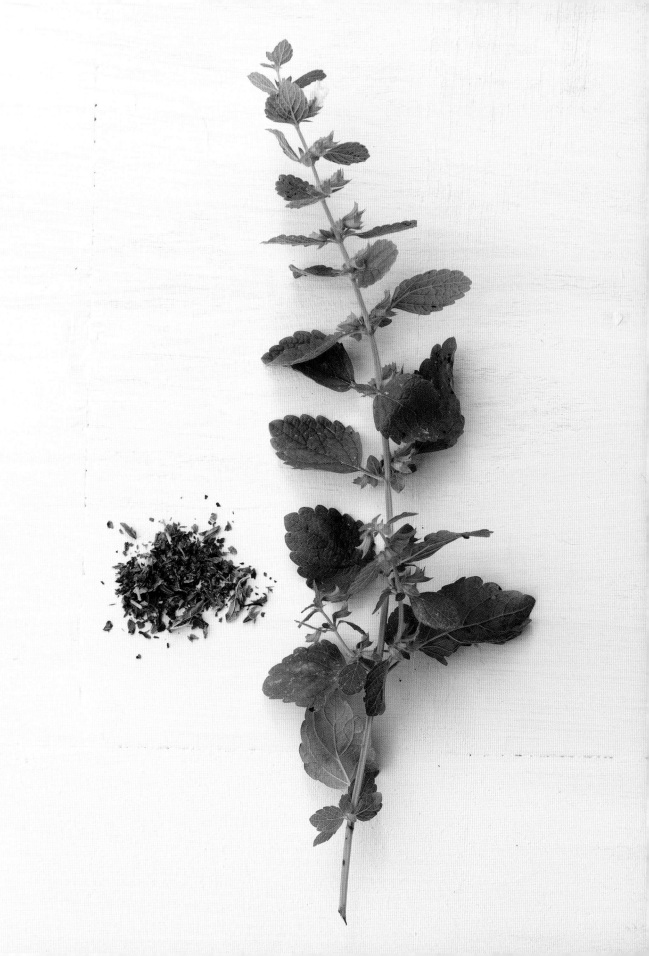

SAGE

(Salvia officinalis)

Think of sage as an antimicrobial and antiseptic powerhouse. Its astringent nature makes it a useful aid with skin infections, lackluster skin, and scalp issues.

Parts used: leaves

Sage is a favorite in the kitchen and the garden, but it can do much more than flavor food. I use sage leaves in my body-care preparations because they have strong antimicrobial and antiseptic properties. The volatile oil is a very effective treatment for many different types of bacteria and fungus, even some that are resistant to antibiotics. Astringent and toning, sage can repair infected skin, clear up acne, and firm up sagging, aging complexions.

Sage is also fantastic for hair. Its astringing qualities strengthen the follicles, which can often result in thicker, fuller hair. Sage can also alleviate itchy scalp and dandruff and darken hair.

Singers who have laryngitis often gargle with sage, as it soothes sore throats. Sage is also good for drying up mucus and phlegm.

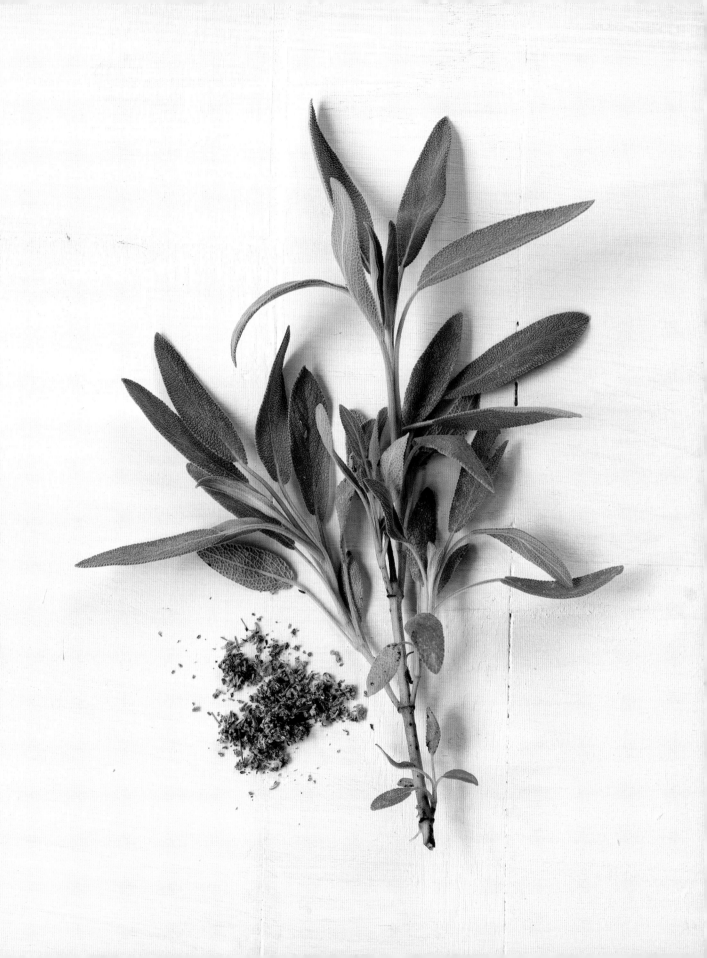

CHICKWEED

(Stellaria media)

Think of this as first aid for your skin, a go-to for minor cuts, wounds, itching, and irritation.

Parts used: leaves, stems, and flowers

I love chickweed! It's one of the first flowers of spring. It always tells me that warmer weather is on the way. An incredibly common plant, chickweed is probably growing in your yard right now.

All of the chickweed's aerial parts—the leaves, stems, and flowers—are useful. Both emollient and demulcent, chickweed can soothe skin that's irritated, inflamed, or dry.

It's especially effective for rashes and for soothing minor cuts, burns, and wounds. Chickweed can also neutralize toxins and comfort environmentally damaged skin. Like aloe, chickweed is great for relieving sunburns.

Chickweed makes a tasty juice. It's delicious in salads and as a green on sandwiches (try it in place of sprouts), and it makes an attractive, bright green pesto.

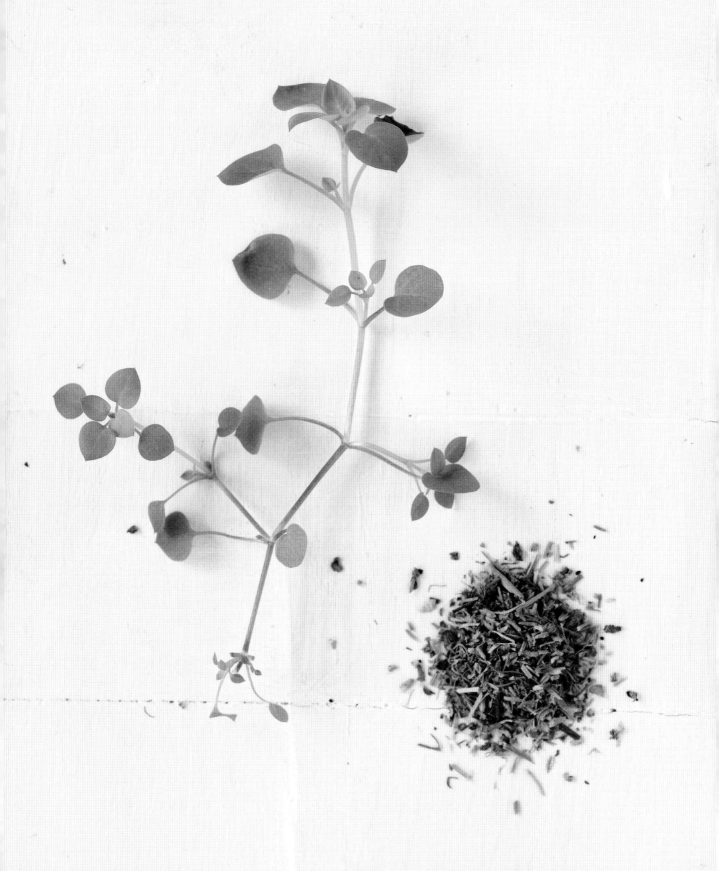

PEPPERMINT

(Mentha piperita)

Peppermint is as cooling and refreshing to the skin as it is to the palate.

Parts used: leaves

We're all familiar with peppermint. You might be growing it in your garden or have it stashed in the pantry as a tea or baking extract. It's very easy to grow. Since it's incredibly yummy, it's often used in teas to mask less pleasant tasting herbs.

The leaves of the peppermint plant can be used for many purposes. Because peppermint is cooling, it's great for soothing inflamed skin and minor burns. Astringent and antiseptic, it can tone and tighten the skin, shrink the appearance of pores, and combat acne. It's especially good for oily to normal skin.

The antiseptic qualities of peppermint make it helpful for killing bacteria that cause undesirable odors and bad breath. It can be used to make a breath-freshening gargle and a deodorizing bath for the body or feet.

Peppermint is also stimulating. It has a refreshing scent that can awaken the mind and make the body feel renewed. A great morning booster, it's also refreshing after a long day.

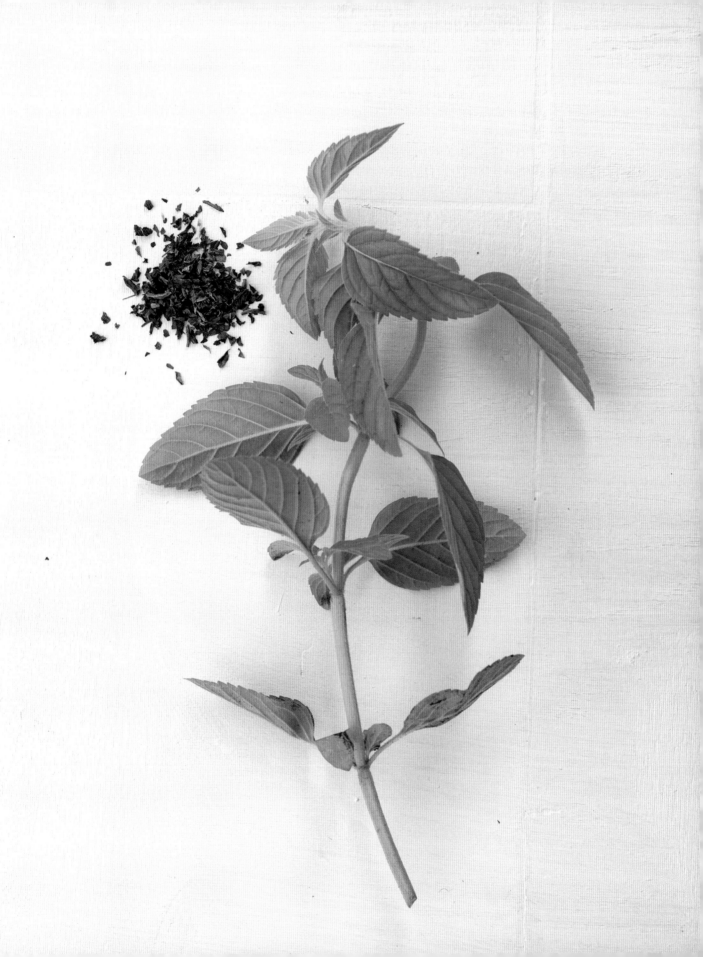

NETTLE

(Urtica dioica)

Also known as "stinging nettles," this highly nutritive plant with its numerous benefits to the body is considered one of the most widely useful herbs. Used both internally and externally, it aids in health, skin, nails, and hair.

Parts used: leaves and stems

A common weed that thrives near water, nettle is one of the easiest plants to identify because it stings! As a result, nettle is harder to harvest than some of our other plant friends. Make sure you wear gloves when you gather it. You want to collect the top of the nettle plant, the stem, and the top 4 inches of the leaves.

Although I use nettle in some of my body-care recipes, it's most useful for skin and hair when ingested. But you need to cook it first to remove the sting! In recipes, it makes a wonderful substitute for spinach, because it's similar in flavor and has far more vitamins and minerals. As a general tonic, there's almost nothing better than nettle. It can act as a diuretic, helping to prevent water retention and reduce bloating. It's an excellent treatment for women with intense PMS and is specifically used to help with heavy bleeding because of its high vitamin K content. Nettle is a bit like a vitamin factory. High in vitamins and minerals, it's one of the best sources of digestible iron, and it contains high levels of calcium, vitamin A, and chlorophyll, helping hair grow longer, thicker, and fuller, and strengthening brittle nails. It has long been used in blood-building and liver tonics. It can enrich the blood and nourish the nervous system, making it the perfect herb for those who suffer from mood swings.

Nettles are also wonderful for the liver and can help the body process toxins internally rather than pushing them out through the skin, which can lead to acne. I've also found that regularly ingesting nettles gives skin a healthy glow.

When used externally, nettles have astringing and toning properties, which means they're a great addition to skin-care products. They can firm up sagging skin and reduce the size of pores. Nettle used externally in hair preparations can improve the health, quality, and appearance of hair. They'll bring out lowlights and darken hair slightly.

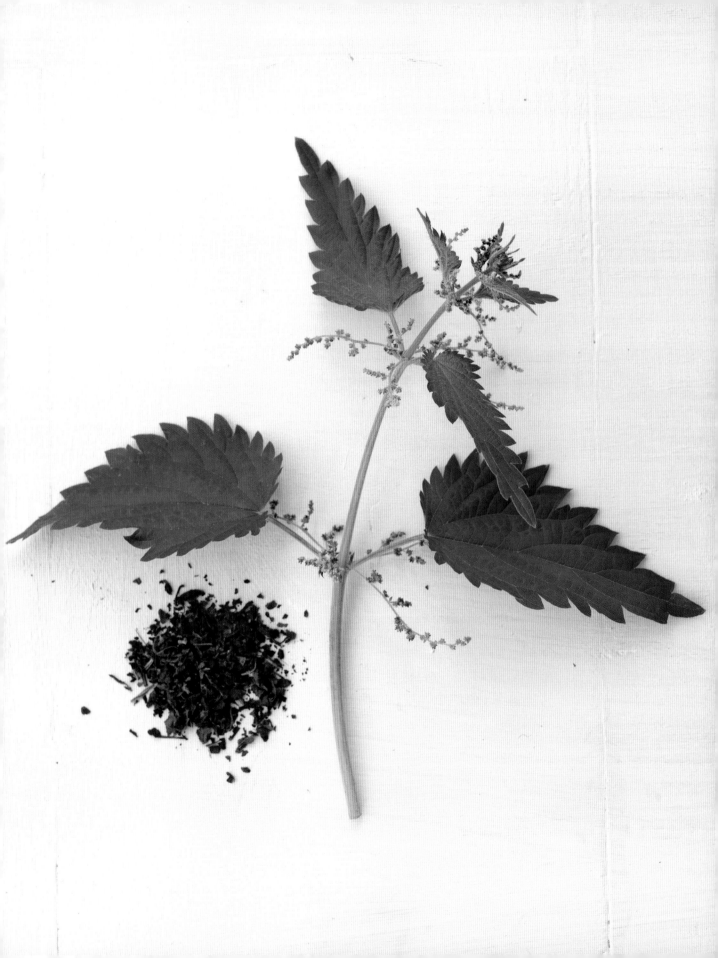

Necessary Tools

All of the recipes in this book can be made using tools that are probably already in your kitchen. Although I know people that keep separate utensils for making body care products, this is unnecessary. Since nothing we're making is toxic, it's safe to use the same kitchen equipment for preparing your food as for making your body care products. Just please make sure everything is as clean as possible to prevent introducing added bacteria that can cause your products to spoil, go rancid, or grow mold.

Some items that are important to have are:

Blender and/or a food processor Although these items aren't interchangeable, I've generally only had one or the other, and I've always been able to make it work with my recipes.

Metal or plastic strainer Either one will work when straining herbs from menstruums.

Measuring cups and measuring spoons You'll use these extensively in almost all the recipes for measuring quantities.

Large mixing bowls These are useful for combining and mixing ingredients.

A pot and makings for a double boiler You'll need these for heating, as well as melting and combining.

Storage containers with lids for your body products These can include: plastic baggies, glass jars, and other storage containers (see the Packaging section on 123 for ideas).

Knives Used for chopping herbs.

Spoons For mixing and stirring.

Eye droppers When you need to dispense small quantities of liquids or fill especially small containers.

Cheesecloth Cheesecloth is perfect for straining plant parts from menstruums.

Grater You'll need a grater for beeswax. The grater is the ONLY tool that you should keep separate from what you use for food. While beeswax is nontoxic, I've found it nearly impossible to get all the beeswax off a grater. So if you don't keep a separate grater for your beeswax, you may find bits of wax in your cheese.

A mortar and pestle or grinder You'll use these to grind herbs. A mortar and pestle can sometimes be tricky to use, and metal hand-cranked grinders work well for grinding small quantities of herbs, but I've found that the easiest way to grind herbs is with an electric coffee grinder. Many people say you must use a separate grinder for herbs than for coffee or your coffee will taste like herbs, and vice versa. However, You can use the same grinder if you run uncooked rice in the grinder between grinding coffee and herbs.

Funnel Various-sized funnels make it easy to dispense products into containers.

Chopsticks These are handy for when you need to poke the air bubbles out of menstruums that you're infusing with herbs.

Stickers or labels It's essential to label your products, not only so you remember what the product is and what it's for, but also so you can list the ingredients and the date you made it.

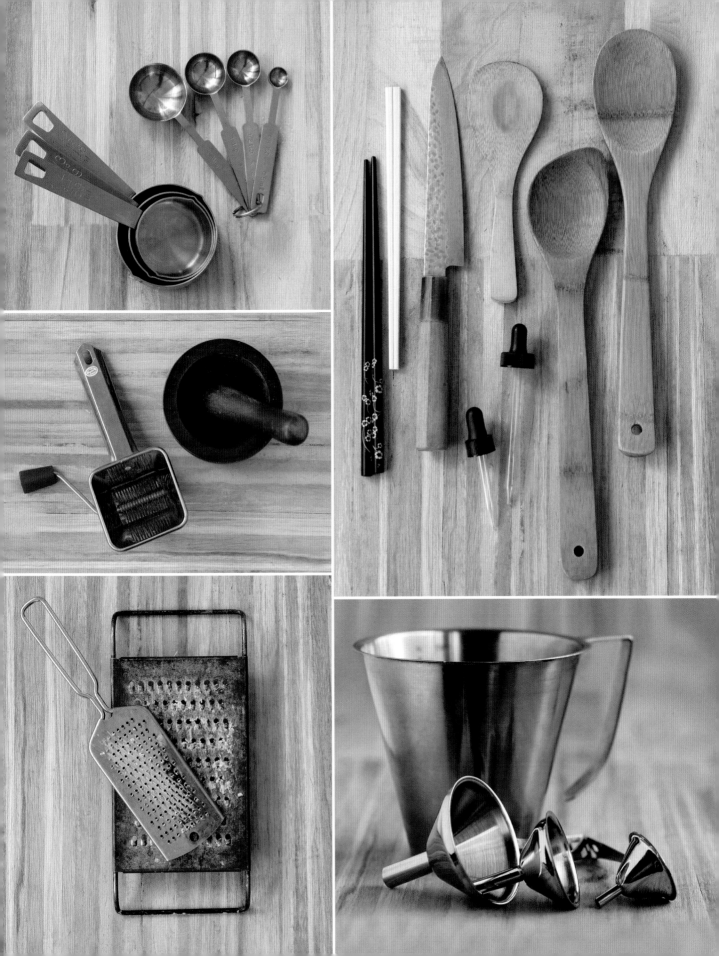

ESSENTIAL ADDITIVES

In addition to plants, many other natural ingredients with healing properties are used in body-care products. These ingredients include oils, honey, beeswax, clays, salts, vitamins, glycerin, water, alcohol, and essential oils.

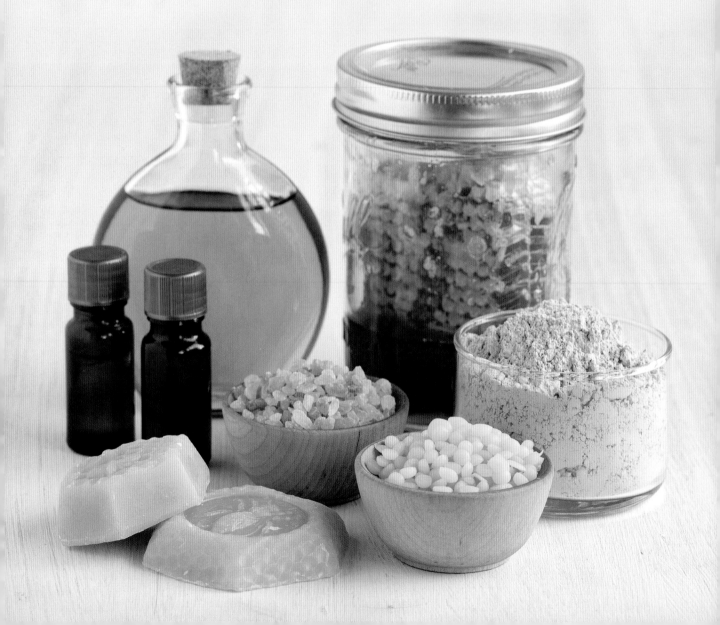

TYPES OF OILS

Oils serve as the basis for many herbal body products, including hair serums, lotions, and cleansers. Oils provide a moist barrier between the skin and hair and the rest of the world. They relieve overly dry skin and hair, and act as an emollient to help both retain their natural elasticity. Nourishing and revitalizing, oils make wonderful cleansers and make-up removers. They're also great for treating brittle nails.

But all oils are not the same! There are basically two types: oils that are solid at room temperature, and oils that are liquid at room temperature. You can personalize your bath and body-care products by choosing oils that will suit your skin and hair type.

Almond
Light and nearly odorless, almond oil can be slightly drying, but it's good for most skin types. It's often mixed with more emollient oils. Because it's especially good for softening the skin, I use it in creams and lotions. **Note:** This oil is often extracted from almonds with solvents, which can be bad for the skin. I use only cold-pressed almond oil in my recipes.

Apricot Kernel
This oil is light and slightly drying. It's good for oily and sensitive skin. It can also be mixed with more emollient oils and used to treat dry skin.

Argon
Argon is a wonderful food for the skin, because it contains many vitamins and fatty acids. It's absorbed quickly and is especially good for damaged, severely dry, and aged skin. Argon can be used to make amazing hot-oil treatments for damaged, brittle hair. It's very expensive, though, so I use it sparingly.

Avocado
Excellent for dry or damaged complexions, this oil is rich, heavy, and penetrating. It's filled with vitamins and essential fatty acids that are beneficial for problem or irritated skin and for scaling skin conditions such as eczema or psoriasis.

Borage Seed
Rich in essential fatty acids and nutritive for the skin, borage-seed oil is a wonderful rejuvenator for aged or damaged complexions. It can help reduce the appearance of scars and wrinkles. It's also a wonderful treatment for acne. Borage-seed oil is very expensive. **Note:** Because the oil can't be heated and must be kept refrigerated, it's unsuitable for some recipes.

Canola
You probably have this common cooking oil in your kitchen. Made from the seeds of the rape plant, canola oil is neutral and light and can be used on most skin types. Because it helps to lock in moisture, it's a great dry-skin treatment, although I've found that it isn't particularly nutritive for damaged skin. On the plus side, it's very inexpensive. To save money, I mix it with other, more expensive nutritive oils.

Cocoa Butter
Made from the fat that's extracted from cocoa beans, this oil has a heavenly chocolate scent. It's solid at room temperature, but it melts when applied to the skin. I use it as an emulsifier and stiffener in creams. It's very protective and helps keep the skin hydrated. It's wonderful for healing overly dry or aged skin and makes a wonderful balm for new tattoos. Because it's somewhat waterproof, cocoa butter is helpful in sunscreens. **Note:** Cocoa butter can be too heavy for some skin types, including oily complexions.

Coconut

One of my all-time favorites for skin, hair, and nails, coconut oil is solid at room temperature, but it melts when applied to the skin or in temperatures that exceed 76°F. A cooling oil that's good for burn creams and salves, it can be used as an emulsifier and thickener in recipes. It's excellent for aged and damaged skin and for sensitive or problem complexions. I've found that coconut oil reduces the appearance of wrinkles and scars. It's extremely emollient but not as heavy as other emollient oils. I find it to be suitable even for oily skin. It makes an excellent oil-conditioning treatment that will leave hair looking thicker and shiny. And it smells amazing!

Flaxseed

Flaxseed oil is very high in omega-3. It's excellent for treating eczema, psoriasis, and other skin conditions. It's also helpful for healing for aged, dry, or damaged skin. *Note:* Because it's unstable and can easily turn rancid, flaxseed oil should be kept refrigerated. It also has a strong odor that can make it unsuitable for some recipes.

Grapeseed

This is one of the lightest oils out there. It's virtually odorless, which means it makes a great carrier oil in perfumes and scented body-care recipes. It absorbs quickly into the skin, although it can be slightly drying. Unless it's mixed with more emollient oils, it isn't suitable for dry skin. I love to use it in lotions and creams because it's smooth but not greasy. It's also good for acne and for problem skin. *Note:* Grapeseed oil can be extracted with solvents that are bad for the skin. You should use the expeller-pressed kind in your recipes.

Jojoba

This oil is made from the seeds of the simmondsia chinensis (jojoba) plant, a small desert shrub with leathery leaves. Technically, it isn't an oil—it's a liquid plant wax. Jojoba resembles human sebum, the natural coating that protects skin and keeps it supple. When applied, it acts like a second skin, providing protection and emolliency while allowing the skin to breathe. It's easily absorbed and excellent for treating aged, dry, and damaged complexions. It's good for acne, too. Stable, with a pleasant, nutty scent, jojoba is helpful as a cleanser in shampoo and great for damaged hair. It's also a good addition to sunscreen products. It's one of my favorite skin-care oils! *Note:* Jojoba oil is indigestible and shouldn't be used for cooking.

Olive

You probably have this one in your kitchen! Used for centuries in the Mediterranean in skin and hair treatments, olive oil contains many beneficial constituents. Heavy, with a somewhat strong smell, it can be used alone or in combination with other oils. It takes a little longer than other oils to be absorbed into the skin, but it's excellent for dry and sensitive complexions. Olive oil can make aged skin seem supple and help reduce the appearance of scars. It can be used to make wonderful hot-oil treatments for hair, and it helps with dandruff.

Peanut

Extracted from peanuts, this oil is rich and heavy, with a strong scent. It penetrates the skin well and is especially good for dry and malnourished complexions. It can be helpful for eczema and other scaling-skin conditions. *Note:* Peanut oil can be susceptible to fungus.

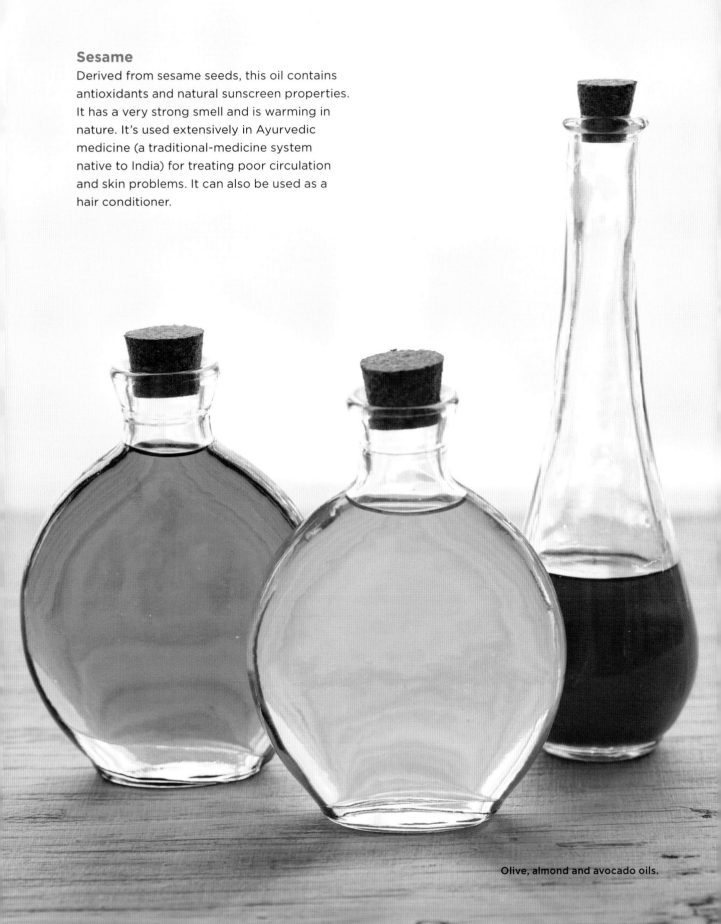

Sesame

Derived from sesame seeds, this oil contains antioxidants and natural sunscreen properties. It has a very strong smell and is warming in nature. It's used extensively in Ayurvedic medicine (a traditional-medicine system native to India) for treating poor circulation and skin problems. It can also be used as a hair conditioner.

Olive, almond and avocado oils.

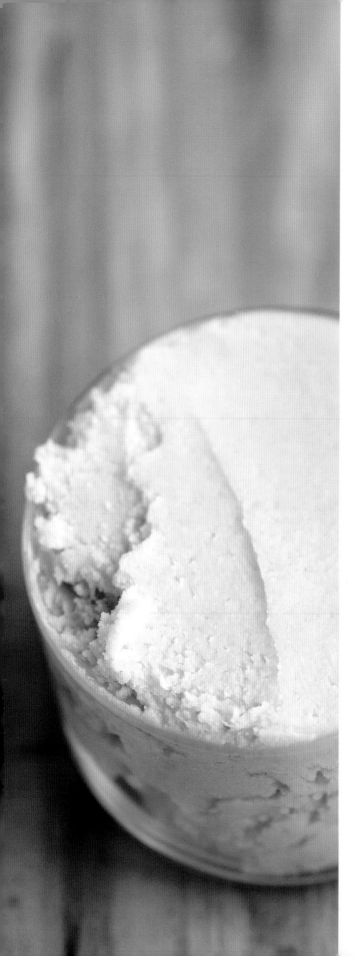

Shea Butter

I love shea butter! It makes the skin feel luxurious, soft, and supple. Therapeutic and healing, it's good for treating dry, aged, and damaged skin. It can provide ultraviolet protection (it has an SPF of 6) and is useful in sunscreens. It contains constituents that help to heal bruises and relieve soreness. It's heavy and penetrating—some people find it too heavy for daily use. It can be a bit pricey, but a little of it goes a long way. Shea butter is solid at room temperature, but it melts on the skin. It can be used as an emulsifier in recipes.

Soy

This relatively inexpensive oil is high in vitamin E and good for healing problem skin. It can help clarify uneven complexions, get rid of blotchiness, and improve aged skin. It's another oil that I mix with more expensive ones in order to cut costs.

Sunflower Seed

This lovely oil contains vitamins A, D, and E, as well as essential fatty acids. It's very therapeutic for malnourished, aged, and dry skin. It can help reduce the appearance of wrinkles and heal cracked or scaling skin. **Note:** This is another oil that may be extracted with harmful chemicals. You should use expeller-pressed sunflower-seed oil in your recipes. Also, this oil is somewhat unstable and thus unsuitable for some recipes. It should be stored in a cool, dark area.

Wheat Germ

Wheat-germ oil is extremely nourishing and contains vitamins A, D, and E. Highly concentrated, with a distinctive nutty smell, it's very therapeutic for cracked, rough skin. It's also great for reducing the appearance of wrinkles.

PRESERVATIVES

Preservatives help to extend the quality and shelf life of body-care preparations. I use several substances as preservatives in my recipes, including honey, beeswax, clay, and salt.

Honey

Honey is the food bees make out of the nectar they gather from flowers. When we think of honey, we usually have in mind the variety that's produced by the genus of bees called Apis. Other insects and other types of bees produce different kinds of honey with very different properties.

Bees make honey as a group through a process of regurgitation and digestion. They remove water from the honey by fanning their tiny wings over it, which causes the water to evaporate. In addition to reducing the honey's water content, this process raises its sugar content. Honey thus contains the perfect water-to-sugar ratio, which means that it won't spoil or ferment if it's properly sealed. Honey does have the ability to absorb water from the air, so it should always be stored properly to prevent fermentation.

I've always been drawn to bees and feel that there's something magical about honey. It has tremendous healing properties. I use it internally and externally.

External Uses

Honey is a mild antiseptic, which makes it a great treatment for wounds, scrapes, and burns. It's anti-inflammatory and analgesic, meaning that it can reduce the pain and swelling that accompany injuries. These properties also make honey a very effective treatment for painful acne outbreaks. Honey promotes the growth of new skin and acts as an exfoliant. It's useful for treating aged, damaged, or dry skin, and chapped lips

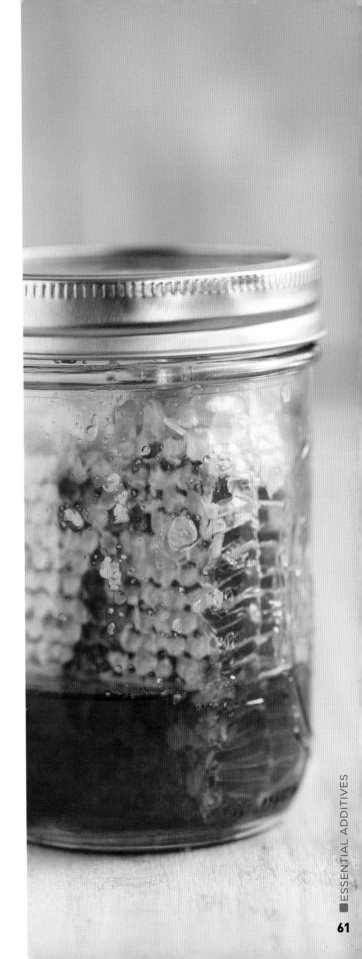

BUYING IN BULK

A friend of mine shared this tip with me: Buy a large quantity of beeswax, melt it down in a double boiler, and pour it into one-ounce molds or ice-cube trays. This makes the measuring process more manageable and makes large quantities of beeswax easier to work with. An added bonus: Buying blocks of bulk beeswax can be cheaper than buying it in smaller quantities.

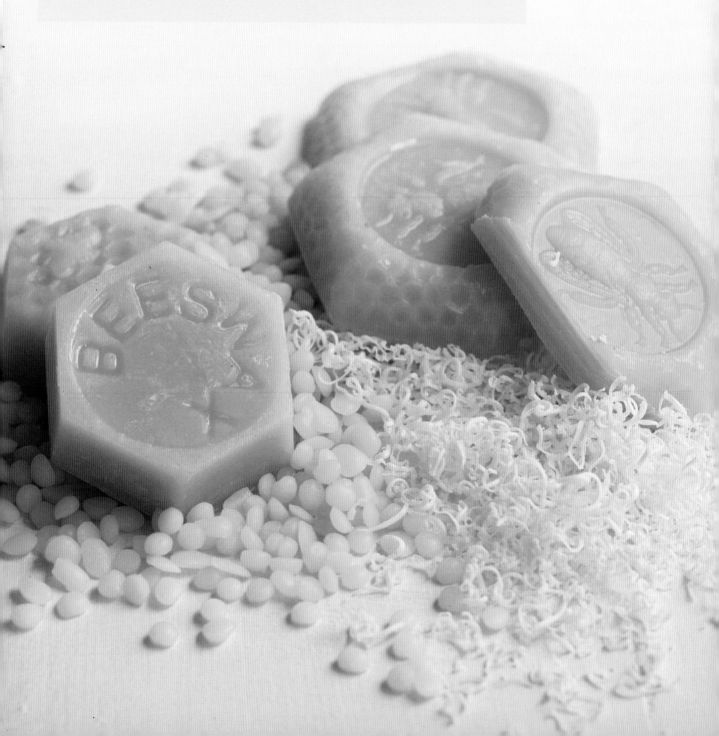

because it actually pulls and binds with moisture from the air. I find that honey makes my skin incredibly soft and gives it a lovely youthful, glow. Additionally, honey is useful in dealing with periodontal disease and mouth ulcers.

Internal Uses

Honey is used internally to help with chronic fatigue and wasting diseases. It can help increase energy, build physical stamina, and improve the immune system. It has a calming effect on the mind and body and can help promote sleep. The antioxidants in honey are thought to reduce the colon damage that occurs with colitis.

Coating and soothing to sore throats, honey can also help with coughs. It's anti-microbial and has amazing wound-healing properties. Honey is also an effective treatment for diabetic ulcers.

Beeswax

Glands in the worker bees of the genus Apis secrete beeswax. Humans have used it for thousands of years. It's a great thickener for salves, creams, lip balms, and lotions. It has preservative and antibacterial properties, which can help extend the shelf life of body-care products, and a warm, appealing, honey-like odor.

Beeswax never goes bad. It can be reheated and reused. It comes in blocks or pellets. The blocks should be grated or cut into very small pieces. The pellets can be used as is. If you don't have a scale, you can eyeball-measure your beeswax. (A tablespoon of pellets is roughly ¼ ounce.) I buy beeswax in 1-ounce blocks; if I need ¼ ounce, I grate about a quarter of the block. I use a cheese grater to grate beeswax, although a potato peeler works well, too. Whatever tool you use, make sure you only use it with beeswax!

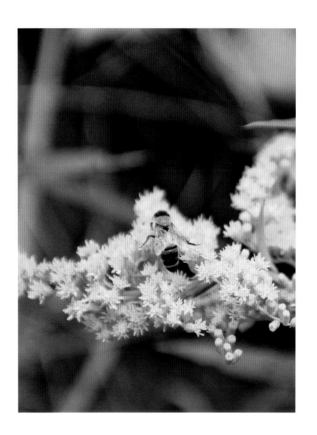

HONEY'S LONG HISTORY

Humans and bees have a long history. Cave paintings in Spain made 8,000 years ago include depictions of bees and of people collecting honey. Traces of honey were found inside clay pots in eastern European gravesites dating back 5,500 years. Ancient Egyptians and Middle Easterners cooked with honey, embalmed their dead with it, and offered it up to their gods and goddesses. In China, the art of beekeeping is so old that no one knows for sure when it started. Honey is mentioned as a medicinal and health food in ancient health texts from India. It was also cultivated in the ancient Americas.

Salt

Another substance with a long cosmetic history, salt contains minerals that are nourishing and is very therapeutic for the skin and hair. It's drawing and detoxifying, excellent as an exfoliator and cleanser. Salt removes toxins, dirt, and dead cells, leaving skin and hair cleaner and softer.

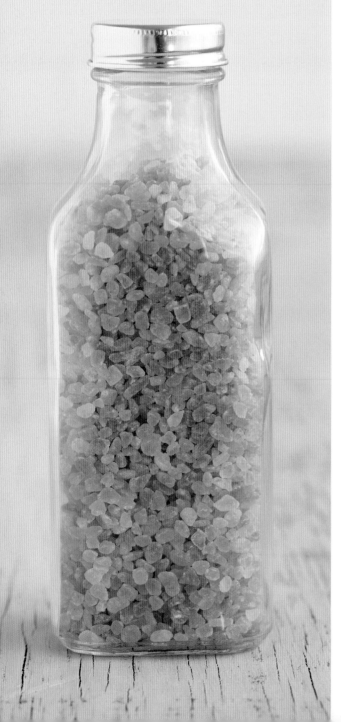

It can help with itchy skin and scalp and remove odors from the body and hair. I find salt soaks to be incredibly relaxing—great for relieving stress and tension. Salt never spoils or goes bad, although humidity may cause it to cake.

There are many different types and colors of salt. Some of my favorites are listed below.

Black Lava Salt

Black lava salt is sea salt that's been mixed with activated charcoal. It contains many trace minerals and is very detoxifying. It's an amazing black-gray color and is very striking when used in bath salts and scrubs, but it can make bath water gray.

Sea Salt

Sea salt is produced when seawater evaporates. Drying and cleansing, abrasive and drawing, it's useful for body scrubs, baths, and hand and foot soaks. Unprocessed sea salt contains more minerals and will be more therapeutic than processed sea salt.

Pink Salt

The color of this salt is caused by its high iron content. Pink salt has a very high percentage of minerals (it contains more than 80 different kinds), which makes it very nourishing for the body. It's very effective at dispelling toxins, and it's great for treating skin issues like psoriasis, eczema, and rashes. A lovely pink color, it can be used to make beautiful floral bath salts and scrubs.

Epsom Salt

Epsom salt isn't really salt! It's a chemical compound that contains magnesium, sulfur, and oxygen. Cleansing and drying, Epsom salt has long been used for cosmetic purposes. It's also valued for its therapeutic, anti-inflammatory properties, which make it helpful for reducing muscle soreness and drawing toxins from the body.

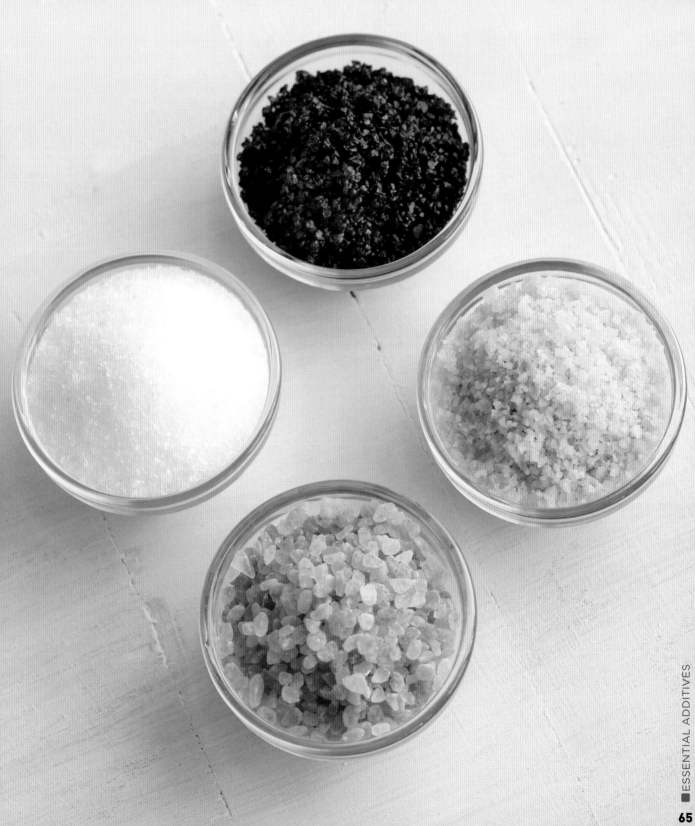

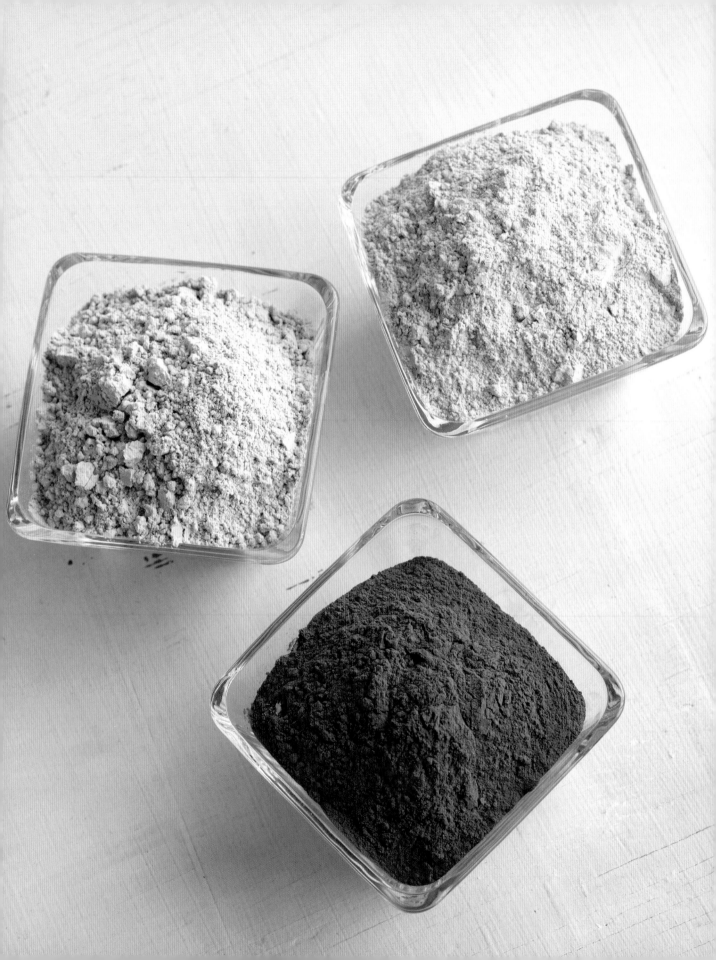

Clay

There's something very primal about using clay on the skin. For thousands of years, clay has served as a cosmetic and as a form of medicine. Packed with minerals and nutrients that nourish the skin, clay has drawing and firming qualities that reduce the appearance of pores and wrinkles. Clay pulls excess oil, dirt, and toxins from the skin and exfoliates dead cells. I find that it leaves my face feeling soft and gives it a youthful glow.

There are many different kinds of clay. The colors and properties of each are determined by the minerals they contain. Different clays are suitable for different skin types.

Bentonite

This soft, mucilaginous clay results from the weathering of volcanic ash. It's mild and good for all skin types, especially problem skin. I find it to be very healing.

Green Clay

Sometimes called sea clay, this clay contains high concentrations of decomposed plant material, which give it a green color. It's mild and compatible with most skin types. It's my favorite clay to use in face masks.

Red Clay

The iron in this clay gives it a distinctive rust color. Extremely detoxifying, red clay is a drying, drawing substance, which makes it perfect for people with acne, oily complexions, or problem skin. I like to use this clay in treatments for poison ivy and poison oak.

White Clay

Also known as kaolin, white clay is the least drying of all the clays. It's incredibly mild and best suited to dry or irritated skin. Because it's safe for all skin types, white clay is widely used in recipes. It has a satiny texture and feels very luxurious.

Other Common Preservatives

One of the chemical elements found in commercial body products are preservatives. While most natural products will have a limited shelf life, there are some preservative elements we can add to help prolong that shelf life. Luckily, these elements also have additional therapeutic effects, which can add to the healing quality of our homemade body care products.

Vitamin E

Vitamin E helps prevent oil-based body products from going rancid. High in antioxidants that repair and protect the skin, vitamin E also helps reduce fine lines and wrinkles.

Vegetable Glycerin

This clear, odorless compound of carbon, hydrogen, and oxygen is obtained from plants through a complicated extraction method called hydrolysis that involves pressure, heat, and water. Vegetable glycerin has a sweet flavor and a syrup-like consistency. It's useful internally and externally. It's often substituted for alcohol in recipes for the herbal extracts known as tinctures.

Vegetable glycerin is very emollient and hydrating for the skin. It hydrates by pulling moisture up from the lower layers of skin, and it also draws moisture from the air. It's soothing for dry complexions, as well as sensitive and problem skin. If it's stored in a cool, dark area, it will keep for a couple of years.

Alcohol

I use alcohol in my body-care products because it has antiseptic and preservative qualities. I also use it to make tinctures.

I use alcohol sparingly because it can dry and irritate the skin. However, it makes an excellent preservative, and a little of it goes a very long way. When I need a preservative or am making a tincture, I typically use vodka. I sometimes use rubbing alcohol to make liniments that are for external use only.

Distilled Water

I use distilled water when making my body-care products. Even when it's filtered, tap water may contain bacteria, fungi, and other substances that can cause the products to spoil or go rancid. Distilled water is relatively inexpensive, and I've found that it does make a difference in the shelf life of my cosmetics.

ESSENTIAL OILS

Essential oils are concentrated plant extracts obtained most often by distillation from flowers, roots, leaves, bark, or peel. I often add essential oils to salves, herbal oils, and lotions. They make the products smell wonderful and can enhance their therapeutic value. Essential oils are strongly antimicrobial and can function as preservatives in cosmetics.

They're also very volatile, meaning that they evaporate quickly and easily into the air. As a result, they should be kept in tightly lidded containers and stored in a cool, dark place. Most essential oils are so concentrated that they're only safe for external use. And most of them need to be diluted before they're applied to the skin. In my opinion, lavender and tea-tree essential oils are the only ones that are safe to use undiluted.

Essential oils can transform our emotional, mental, and physical states. I love to use them in my body-care products. A few of my favorites are listed on the following page.

Bergamot *(Citrus bergamia)*

This essential oil is used to flavor Earl Grey tea. Its warm, spicy, citrusy scent is one of my favorites for use in cosmetics. Bergamot oil refreshes, balances, and helps to ease anxiety, nervous tension, and depression. ***Note:*** Bergamot oil may cause photosensitivity in people with very light skintone. Pregnant women should avoid the oil because its effects on unborn children are not known. People with disorders like epilepsy should also avoid bergamot oil, because it could induce seizures.

Citrus oils *(Citrus spp)*

Oils like lemon, orange, and lime are all related to bergamot. They're relatively inexpensive. Sweet-scented, uplifting, and invigorating, citrus oils are wonderful mood-balancers. Because they're astringent and disinfecting, they're great for treating acne and balancing out combination skin.

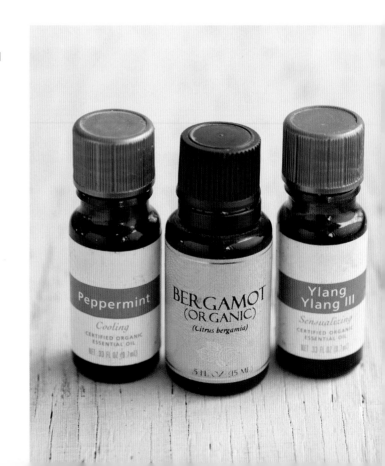

Clary sage (*Salvia sclarea*)

Clary sage has long been used in the making of cosmetics. Known as an aphrodisiac and a mood booster, this lovely oil has a warm, musky, floral scent. It's antimicrobial and astringent. A helpful treatment for acne, it calms inflamed skin and can restore balance to oily complexions and oily hair. Clary sage is also great for treating dandruff. ***Note:*** Like bergamot, this essential oil should be avoided during pregnancy.

Eucalyptus (*Eucalyptus globulus*)

This essential oil has strong antimicrobial and expectorant properties. Used in inhalation therapy to treat upper-respiratory ailments, it's cooling, refreshing, and stimulating. It can also be used as a deodorant and is effective as a bug repellent.

Frankincense (*Boswellia carterii*)

I love the smell of this essential oil. I think it has an air of mystery and timelessness. Made from the resin of an endangered tree that grows in the Middle East, frankincense has been used for thousands of years and is known to reduce stress, anxiety, and tension. It can also rejuvenate tired, sagging skin, reduce wrinkles, and heal blemishes and small wounds. I find it to be wonderful treatment for acne and for skin that's environmentally damaged or mature.

Lavender (*Lavendula spp*)

One of my favorite essential oils because it's safe to use and effective in such a wide variety of ways, lavender is in a class by itself. It's one of the few essential oils that can be applied to the skin safely with no dilution. Its piney-floral scent soothes the nervous system, alleviates stress, and acts as a mild antidepressant. Relaxing and calming, it's a great remedy for insomnia. It's also very effective for relieving headaches (I've eased many a terrible headache by simply rubbing a little lavender oil on my temples). The oil is excellent for all skin types and can help to treat a myriad of skin problems, from acne to burns and bug bites. Its antimicrobial, anti-inflammatory, and regenerative properties make it helpful for improving aged skin, fighting acne, and restoring balance to the complexion. It's also relatively inexpensive.

Myrrh (*Commiphora myrrha*)

Another ancient resin oil from the Middle East, myrrh was used by the ancient Egyptians to embalm mummies. It has a deep, earthy scent. It's very antimicrobial and can be applied to cuts, scrapes, and bug bites to prevent infection and assist with healing. I often use it as a preservative in my lotions, creams, and salves. It can act as a deodorizer, and it has astringent, anti-inflammatory properties that make it a helpful treatment for acne and for oily complexions.

Tea Tree (*Melaleuca alternifolia*)

Potent yet safe, tea tree oil has a crisp, clean scent. It's antibacterial, antifungal, and antiviral. I've seen it do wonders as an acne treatment. It's also helpful for healing wounds, cuts, infections, and rashes. Tea tree oil works well in cleaners and astringents and can be used directly on the skin without being diluted. It makes a wonderful spot treatment for pimples.

Ylang Ylang (*Canangium odoratum*)

Sweet and floral, the scent of ylang ylang is one of my favorites. Ylang Ylang inspires feelings of well-being and is traditionally used in aphrodisiac and euphoric formulas. A moderate antiseptic, it's a good remedy for oily skin. It also helps promote skin-cell growth and can reduce the appearance of scars and wrinkles.

Substitutions

In the long run, making your own body-care products is significantly cheaper than buying ready-made items at the drugstore. Dollar-wise, though, your initial investment may seem considerable. But I've found that the ingredients I purchase for making my own products are enough to produce large or multiple batches.

I'm no stranger to thrift and have discovered some smart ways to cut down on costs. Here are a few money-saving ideas:

→ Oils, especially the very nourishing, luxurious ones, tend to be pricey. If the recipe I'm making calls for an especially expensive oil such as borage or argon, I'll cut the amount I use in half and compensate with a cheaper substitute like avocado, grapeseed, or canola oil. For instance, if I'm making a cream that requires one cup of borage oil, I may use a half-cup of borage and a half-cup of a less expensive oil.

→ Eliminate those expensive oils altogether and do total substitutions. Just because an oil is expensive doesn't necessarily mean it's better! I find some of the less expensive oils to be just as effective as the pricey ones.

→ Share, share, share! You'll often get a better deal if you buy large quantities of items, so go in with friends and split the costs. Have a product-making party. These can be so much fun! I had one recently: my friends and I made products to give as gifts at a wedding.

Although we spent around $100 on supplies, we made adorable facial-product gift bags for nine women, which means we spent only about $12 apiece—significantly cheaper than if we'd purchased ready-made products.

→ Substitute cheaper salts for the more expensive ones. Try using Epsom instead of sea salt.

→ When I need alcohol for a recipe, I use a fairly cheap brand of vodka. Vodka is colorless and doesn't have as profound a taste as other spirits.

→ Essential oils are one of the biggest investments you'll make for your bath and beauty recipes. The little vials of oil do cost a lot! But keep in mind that a very small amount of essential oil goes a long way, so you're investing in ingredients that you'll use to make many batches. You may be tempted to purchase every beautiful, romantic-smelling oil you come across, but if you're trying to economize, I suggest that you invest in a couple of scents that you really, really like. Lavender is a great investment because it's so versatile and cheaper than many other essential oils.

Essential oils make a great group investment if you have people to them share with. My friends and I buy different scents and trade when we want to try different ones. Because many essential oils are simply too big of an investment, I've learned to find scents that I can use as substitutes. Whenever possible, I suggest substitutes for the recipes in this book.

MENSTRUUMS

A menstruum is any substance that can be infused with the healing properties of herbs. Examples include water, oils, alcohol, honey, and glycerin.

Infusing Menstruums with Herbs

I add to the healing properties of my body-care products by infusing some of their raw ingredients with healing herbs. I choose healing herbs that are appropriate for my skin and hair type. Infusing a menstruum with herbs is an easy process that doesn't take much time.

Which are better to use—fresh or dried herbs? In preparations intended for internal use, I prefer fresh. In most cases, fresh herbs are more potent and hold more healing, medicinal power than dried. For external preparations like body-care products, dried herbs are often more effective. With a few exceptions, all of the recipes in this book use dried herbs.

Try to use the freshest dried herbs possible. The medicinal properties of dried herbs degrade the longer they sit. This degradation occurs even faster when the herbs are exposed to light. I keep my dried herbs in glass jars on a shelf. If I dried them myself, I try to use them within six months to a year. If I bought them from a store (where they'd probably been sitting for a while), I try to use them within three to six months.

Making Herbal Oil

An herbal oil can be made with any of the options listed in the Types of Oils section on page 57. There are two different ways to make an herbal oil: through sun infusion and through stove infusion. I prefer the first method because it seems to produce stronger, more potent oils. But if time is tight or you're using a solid oil, the stove-infusion method is the better option. It will definitely give you strong,

healing herbal oils. Also, the stove-infusion method seems to work better with roots, seeds, or woody herbs—substances that don't extract or give up their properties easily.

Method 1: Sun Infusion

(1) When it comes to making herbal oils, dried herbs are better to use than fresh. Because oils will spoil and grow mold if they're exposed to excess moisture from fresh plant material, if you use fresh herbs, they should be wilted. You should chop or crush them and then place them in a glass jar. Fill the jar almost to the top, leaving about 2 inches empty. Do not pack the jar tightly. Make sure there are no air holes in the jar where the oil cannot get to the plant matter.

(2) Pour the oil of your choice over the herbs, making sure you cover them completely. Fill up the jar with oil, leaving a $1/2$ inch of empty space at the top for air. Make sure no plant material protrudes from the oil, as this can cause mold to grow and spoil the mixture.

(3) Press the herbs down with a chopstick or skewer. Make sure there are no air bubbles in the oil.

(4) Put the herbal oil on a sunny windowsill or out in the garden. The sun will warm the oil and release the medicinal properties of the herbs.

(5) Leave the oil in the sun for two weeks. You'll want to shake it occasionally (I shake mine every day to mix the plants around). The agitation helps infuse the oil with the plant properties and ensures there aren't any air bubbles in the oil. It's also a good way to make sure there's no plant material protruding from the oil.

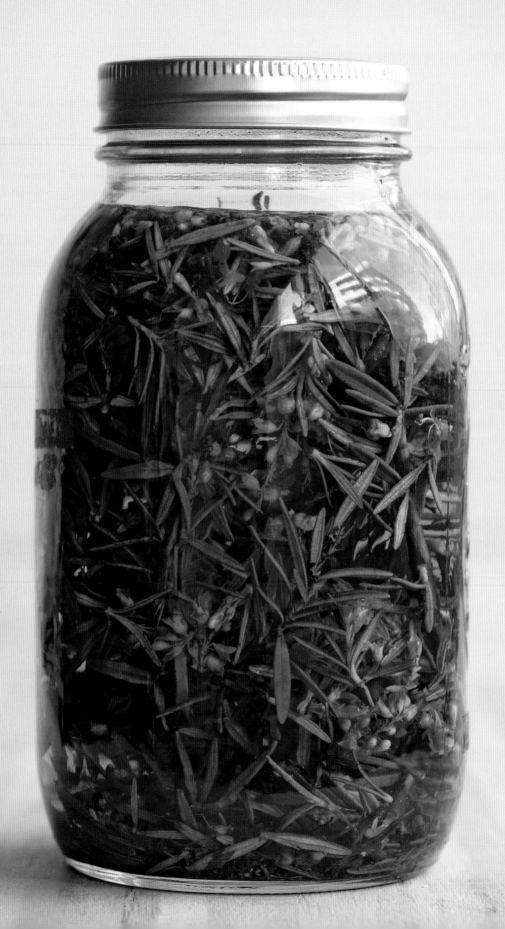

I check my oil each day (I like interacting with it!) and note the changes that occur in its color as the plant matter infuses into it.

(6) Carefully strain all the plant matter from the oil. You can use a plastic or metal mesh strainer, although I find that cheesecloth is more effective. Pour the oil through the strainer two or three times so that as much plant material (including small sediment particles) as possible is removed from the oil.

Method 2: Stove Infusion

(1) Put 4 cups of the oil of your choice in a pot on the stove and warm it over low heat. Aim for about 100°F. You want to warm it, but you definitely don't want to cook or boil it. If you're using a solid oil that's at room temperature, give it time to melt completely. (*Note:* Some people use crockpots to make herbal oils. These are also effective; just make sure the temperature stays around 100°F.)

(2) Chop or crush the herb of your choice (make sure it's wilted). Then add 2 cups of it to the pot of oil.

(3) Allow the oil to sit for 2 to 4 hours. Keep an eye on it and stir it occasionally. It will begin to change color and take on the smell of the herb you added. The longer the oil sits on the stove, the more potent it will be.

(4) Using a mesh strainer or piece of cheesecloth, carefully strain all of the plant matter from the oil (see Straining Plant Matter, right). If you're using a solid oil and it begins to harden during the straining process, you should reheat it.

Transfer the oil to a glass bottle or jar with a lid. Be sure you label and date the container. The oil should be stored in a cool, dark place. If stored properly, it should keep for three to six months—maybe longer. *Note:* You should always check an herbal oil for rancidity before you use it.

STRAINING PLANT MATTER

A plastic or metal strainer can be used to remove plant material from a liquid substance. You may want to strain the mixture two or three times to make sure you get the plant bits out. Make sure you get as much of them out as possible because they can mold and cause your product to spoil more quickly.

Cheesecloth works wonders as a strainer. Here's my method: I secure a square of the material (usually folded into three layers) over the top of my jar with a rubber band. Then I pour the liquid into the jar. The cheesecloth catches the remaining plant material. To get all of the goodness out of that material, I squeeze the cheesecloth over the container. I typically repeat this step a couple of times. You can also use a strainer first and follow up with cheesecloth.

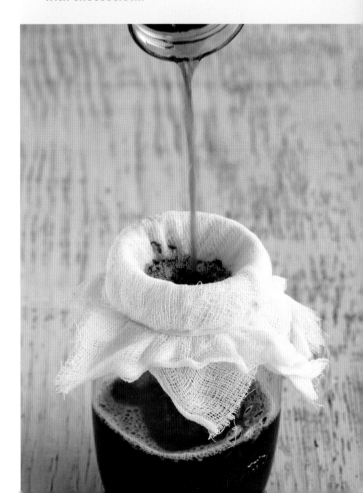

Tinctures

As I mentioned before, a tincture is an alcohol extract of a plant's medicinal properties. A great way to preserve herbs—especially fresh herbs—a tincture is very potent. A small amount (sometimes only a drop) can be very effective.

Tinctures are useful both internally and externally. They're one of the most popular methods of taking herbs internally in the United States. For the purposes of this book, though, we'll only discuss the external uses of tinctures.

Tinctures can be used externally as wound washes, facial toners, and muscle rubs. You can make a tincture in rubbing alcohol that's for external use only. This type of tincture is called a liniment.

The best tinctures are made from fresh herbs. Where many herbs are concerned, tinctures are a great alternative to drying. Freshly dried herbs only retain their potency for a year or so, while tinctures last much longer. Many retain their potency for up to 10 years. As you can see, a little bit of plant material can produce a lot of medicine that will last for a long time.

Tinctures can also be made with dried herbs, although they're sometimes less potent than those made from fresh herbs. Dried-herb tinctures work best with barks, roots, resinous herbs, some berries, and thick, leathery leaves.

In many cases, glycerin can be used instead of alcohol to make tinctures. But keep in mind that certain herbal alkaloids and resins can only be extracted in alcohol or are best extracted in alcohol. An extract made from glycerin is called a glyceride.

Using Alcohol in Tinctures

To make tinctures, herbalists often use a complicated, scientific method involving alcohol percentages and a specific herb-to-alcohol ratio. This method works wonderfully. For the purposes of this book, however, we'll be using a simplified technique that I find to be very effective.

With the simplified method, you can use any liquor or spirit that's 80 to 100 proof. This creates a solution that's 40 to 50% alcohol and capable of extracting the properties of most plants. I use vodka in my tinctures because it's clear and almost tasteless. Some herbalists prefer brandy.

To make a tincture with alcohol following this easy method, here's what you do:

1. Chop up your plant material until it's coarse, and discard anything that's damaged or unusable. You don't need to wash the material.

2. Fill a jar (any size will do) with the plant parts, leaving about 2 inches of empty space at the top.

3. Pour the alcohol over the herbs, making sure you cover them completely. Fill up the jar with alcohol, leaving $\frac{1}{2}$ inch of empty space at the top for air.

4. Poke the mixture with a skewer or chopstick, making sure there are no air pockets in it and that no plant parts are protruding from the alcohol.

5. Cap the jar and label it. It should be kept out of direct light but stored in a place where you can taste or observe it as it changes color. Make sure you shake the jar occasionally over the next four to six weeks.

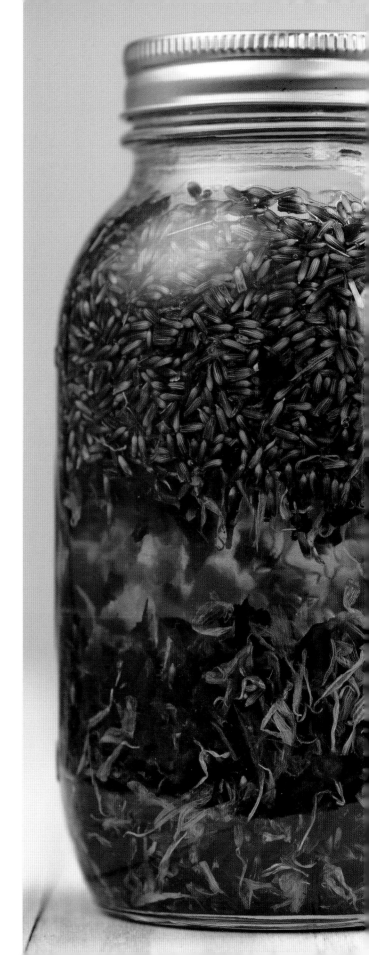

(6) The tincture should be ready to decant and use after four to six weeks but you don't have to strain it right away. I've kept tinctures for months and even years before straining them, and they were incredibly potent. To decant the tincture, pour it through a mesh strainer or a piece of cheesecloth into a new container with a lid. The remaining plant material will contain a lot of alcohol, so transfer it to a piece of cheesecloth and wring the cloth out by hand over the new container. If you're fortunate enough to have a tincture press, the process will be much simpler. You'll also get more of the alcohol out of the plant material.

As a general rule, you'll only tincture one kind of plant per bottle. However, after straining, you can mix tinctures of different plants to create unique blends.

Using Glycerin

Glycerin is excellent to use in external tinctures because of its emollient properties. The method for making a glycerin tincture is the same as the one used for an alcohol tincture—just substitute glycerin for alcohol. A glycerin tincture won't last as long as an alcohol tincture, but if it's stored in a cool, dark spot, it'll be usable for 2 to 3 years.

RECIPES

Our ancient ancestors used plants and other natural substances to care for, clean, and decorate their bodies. We can learn valuable lessons from these distant forebears, who were highly sensitive to their environments and to the natural world. Cosmetic preparations, for them, were more than just a source of adornment. They also served to protect the body from harsh external conditions.

Some of the cosmetic preparations they used would be considered suspect by modern standards, but many of them are similar to the ones we make and depend on today. For instance, the ancient Egyptians used a mixture of frankincense, wax, moringa oil, and fermented plant juice to make a wrinkle-fighting agent that could be applied daily. Fast-forward a few thousand years, and those of us who want to make natural, nourishing body-care products are still relying on essential oils, waxes, and alcohols.

This chapter features a selection of my favorite recipes. From soothing salves and balms to luxurious hair-care and facial products, these are the tried and tested formulas that I turn to the most. Some of them I picked up in herb school, and some I arrived at through my own process of experimentation. Others are adaptations of very old recipes or ideas that were contributed by friends. Many of them are works in progress that I continue to tweak.

Think of these recipes as templates. When it comes to personalizing them, you have many options! I find that experimentation is one of the most exciting parts of making body-care products. Where these recipes are concerned, there are no hard and fast rules. In many cases, the measurements don't even have to be exact. I encourage you to make each one of them a couple of times according to my instructions. Then feel free to experiment with different ratios, scents, oils, and salts. Follow your instincts and indulge your personal taste—whether it be a love for lavender or a preference for tea tree—and make each product your own. Experiment until you arrive at a recipe that's right for you.

When experimenting, make sure you jot down any changes you introduce to a recipe. That way, you'll remember what NOT to do if a product turns out badly. And, of course, a little note-taking will also help you remember what you did right. Trust me—I learned this the hard way. Take good notes!

I also recommend that you gather all of the necessary materials and ingredients before you begin a recipe. It's annoying and inconvenient to have to run out and grab something once a project is underway.

Finally—and most importantly—have fun!

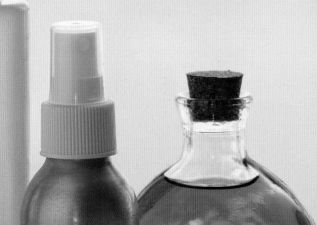

FIRST AID

Everyone gets cuts, scrapes, and burns on occasion. Many of the common first aid products we purchase have great homemade natural alternatives, which are often cheaper and safer than the store-bought versions.

SALVES AND BALMS

Usually medicinal in nature, salves can be used as soothing, healing balms for minor wounds, burns, and muscle aches. They're fun and surprisingly easy to put together.

BASIC SALVE

YOU WILL NEED:

- ½ CUP OIL OR HERB-INFUSED OIL (SEE MAKING HERBAL OIL, PAGE 71)
- SAUCEPAN OR POT
- ¼ OUNCE BEESWAX, GRATED (BEESWAX MAKES THE SALVE HARD. THE MORE OF IT YOU USE, THE HARDER YOUR SALVE WILL BE. EXPERIMENT UNTIL YOUR SALVE IS THE DESIRED CONSISTENCY.)
- SPOON FOR STIRRING
- ROOM-TEMPERATURE SPOON FOR TESTING SALVE
- ¼ TEASPOON VITAMIN E OIL (OPTIONAL)
- 20 TO 40 DROPS ESSENTIAL OIL OF YOUR CHOICE (OPTIONAL)
- SEVERAL CONTAINERS WITH LIDS

(1) Pour the herb-infused or plain oil into the saucepan and set your measuring cup aside (you'll need it later). Warm the oil over very low heat. Make sure it doesn't come anywhere close to simmering.

(2) Add the grated beeswax to the oil, and stir until the beeswax melts.

(3) Test the consistency of the salve. See the tip box below for instructions on how to do this.

(4) Take the pot off the heat and pour the oil back into your measuring cup. Add the vitamin E oil and the essential oil, and stir.

(5) Pour the salve into the containers and cover them. Allow the salve to set and harden before you try it.

TESTING THE CONSISTENCY OF SALVES

The amount of beeswax that you use will determine the consistency of your salve. This is also the case with the other recipes in this book that call for beeswax, including chapstick and some lotions. Checking the texture of a salve or other product is easy. You should check it once the beeswax has melted into the oil, while the oil is still on the heat. Do this by dipping a room-temperature spoon into the mixture and putting the spoon in the fridge for about a minute so that the mixture can cool and harden. Then take the spoon out of the fridge and see how you like it. If the salve in the spoon seems too runny, add a little more beeswax to the oil and wait for it to melt. If the salve seems too hard, add a little more oil to the pot. Repeat until you're satisfied with the salve's consistency.

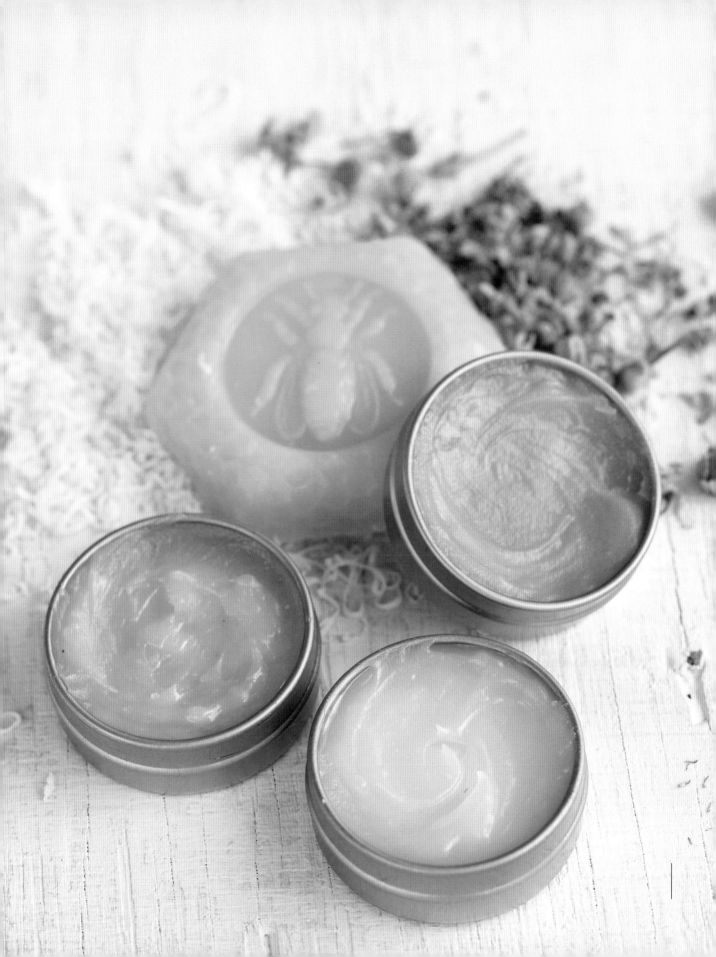

Some of my favorite salve recipes are featured below. Feel free to experiment with the liquid and essential oils you use in these formulas (except for the Eucalyptus and Icy-Hot Salves—their power lies in the essential oils I suggest in the recipes). Be creative and try out some substitutions!

ST. JOHN'S WORT BURN SALVE

This salve is wonderful for minor burns and sunburns. To make it, follow the Basic Salve recipe on page 78. For the herb-infused oil portion of the recipe, use St. John's wort. For the essential oil portion, use 30 drops of lavender.

COMFREY WOUND SALVE

This salve is a terrific wound healer, great for treating minor cuts and burns. It has an antiseptic quality, and it encourages the growth of new skin tissue. It does the trick on sprains and bruises. I used it when I had a broken toe, and it worked wonders. *Note:* I like to infuse my comfrey in olive oil, which can help reduce the appearance of scars.

To make the Comfrey Wound Salve, follow the Basic Salve recipe on page 78. For the herb-infused oil portion of the recipe, use 3½ ounces of comfrey and ½ ounce of chickweed. For the essential-oil portion, use 5 drops of myrrh, 5 drops of tea tree, and 10 drops of lavender.

ICY-HOT FOOT SALVE

I developed this salve as a treatment for my own tired, achy feet. Be warned: It's potent. Some people find it too strong!

To make the Icy-Hot Foot Salve, follow the Basic Salve recipe on page 78. Use plain grapeseed oil or canola oil instead of the herbal-infused oil in this case. You can also try

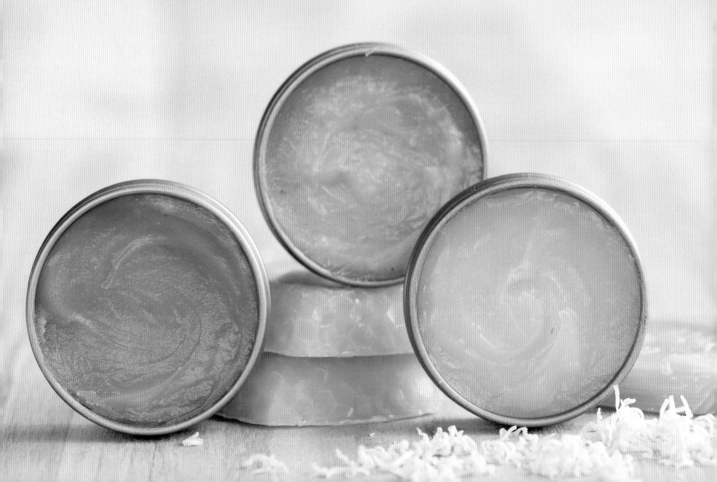

a more emollient oil like avocado or wheat germ, both of which are great for dry feet. The power of this salve lies in the essential oils that are used: add 25 drops of ginger and 25 drops of peppermint essential oil. Feel free to experiment with different herb-infused oils—they'll boost the healing qualities of the product.

EUCALYPTUS SINUS SALVE

A wonderful salve that clears the sinuses and calms coughs, this one is great for the entire family. I use it to treat colds and flu. It works like magic when rubbed on the chest.

To make the Eucalyptus Sinus Salve, follow the Basic Salve recipe on page 78. I typically use plain grapeseed oil instead of the herbal-infused oil in this salve, as it's relatively unscented. For the essential-oil portion of the recipe, use 50 drops of eucalyptus—that's where the power of this product lies. *Note:* If you're making the salve as a treatment for a child, cut the amount of essential oil used in half.

ARNICA SALVE FOR PAIN AND BRUISES

An all-around wonderful salve for pain. I use it on bruises, sprains, and achy muscles.

To make the Arnica Salve for Pain and Bruises, follow the Basic Salve recipe on page 78. For the herb-infused oil portion of the recipe, use arnica. For the essential-oil portion, use 15 drops of clary sage and 10 drops of lavender.

SLEEPY BABY BALM

This relaxing balm is just right for a baby or young child. A little of it goes a long way. A pea-sized amount is all you need to soothe baby's tummy, legs, and feet. This balm is especially nice for colicky infants and can be used to relax tense muscles. It's also soothing for adults and older children.

FOR CHILDREN

These recipes are safe—even for young children. Keep in mind, though, that kids have more sensitive skin than adults. A number of wonderful herbs (including lavender, calendula, and chamomile) are perfectly harmless when used in products for children, but you should use caution when choosing additives and herbs for the recipes you make for youngsters. Clays can sometimes be too drying for young skin, while oils like shea or cocoa butter may be too heavy.

I also suggest that you reduce the amount of essential oils used in the products you make for children. The smell can be overwhelming to kids—too strong for their skin and hair. Remember, too, that essential oils add a preservative quality to body products, which means they may spoil more quickly. A final word of caution: If you're making a product for a child that calls for an alcohol extract, try reducing the amount of alcohol and increasing the amount of water in the recipe.

To make the Sleepy Baby Balm, follow the Basic Salve recipe on page 78, using chamomile-infused herbal oil. I use only 1/8 ounce of beeswax in this balm. As a result, it won't be as hard as the other preparations you've made. In fact, it may seem a bit loose in comparison. For the essential-oil portion of the recipe, add 5 drops of lavender. *Note:* If you're making the balm for an adult or older child, increase the amount of essential oil to 20 drops.

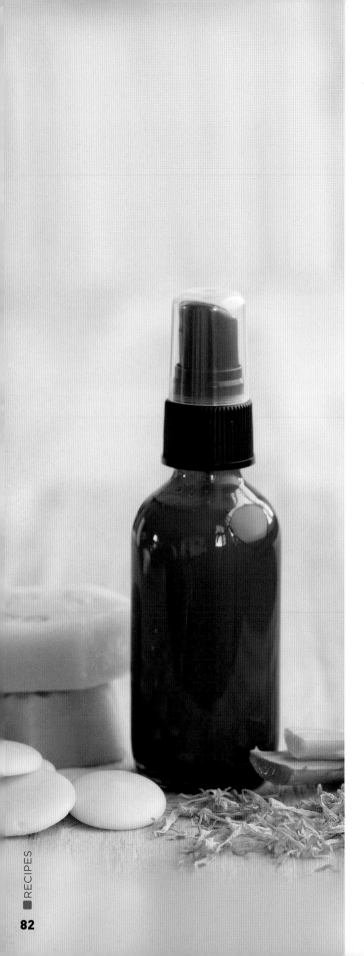

SUNSCREEN

Rich, protective, and nourishing, this all-natural sunscreen is easy to make. With an SPF that falls somewhere in between 4 and 8, it's probably not strong enough for a day at the beach, but it provides perfect coverage for a walk or a meal at an outdoor café.

YOU WILL NEED:

- ¾ OUNCE BEESWAX
- ½ CUP COCONUT OIL
- ¼ CUP COCOA BUTTER
- ¼ CUP SHEA BUTTER
- ⅛ CUP JOJOBA OIL
- ½ CUP SESAME OIL
- ½ CUP CALENDULA INFUSED OIL
- ¼ CUP ALOE VERA GEL
- POT OR SAUCEPAN
- CONTAINER WITH LID
- 50 DROPS ESSENTIAL OIL OF YOUR CHOICE (AVOID BERGAMOT!)

(1) Combine all of the ingredients except for the aloe vera gel and the essential oils in a clean pot.

(2) Heat the mixture on the stove until the beeswax has melted.

(3) Remove the mixture from the heat and add the aloe vera gel. Stir until it's dissolved.

(4) Pour the mixture into a container, add the essential oil, and stir.

BUG REPELLENT

Although they're effective, the commercial bug sprays you find at the drugstore contain potentially harmful chemicals. Luckily, there's an alternative! This all-natural insect repellent uses essential oils to keep those buzzing pests at bay. The spray is easy to make, effective, and (unlike most repellents) it smells terrific.

YOU WILL NEED:

- ½ CUP DISTILLED WATER
- ½ CUP WITCH HAZEL EXTRACT
- 1 TEASPOON GLYCERIN (OPTIONAL)
- 8-OUNCE SPRAY BOTTLE
- 75 DROPS TOTAL OF THESE ESSENTIAL OILS: CITRONELLA, CEDAR, ROSEMARY, EUCALYPTUS, LAVENDER, AND LEMON (IF YOU DON'T HAVE ALL OF THESE ESSENTIAL OILS, USE A COMBINATION OF THE ONES LISTED THAT YOU DO HAVE.)

(1) Pour the water, the witch hazel, and the glycerin into the spray bottle.

(2) Add the essential oils, and cap the bottle. Shake the mixture well before you try it out on the front porch or patio.

HAIR CARE

Although we don't often think of it in these terms, hair is a biomaterial composed largely of protein. It grows from the follicles in our dermis. One of the defining characteristics of mammals, it regulates body temperature, provides protection, and helps with our sense of touch.

Hairstyles and treatments have varied wildly from era to era and culture to culture. In many ancient civilizations, it was customary to pluck or shave all hair from the body. A typical woman in ancient Egypt shaved her head and wore a wig, which served as both a fashion statement and as a precaution against lice and other environmental problems.

Today, many of us think of our hair—long or short, blonde or brunette—as our crowning glory. We express ourselves through the colors and cuts we choose. Given the importance that's placed on hair in our culture, it's unfortunate that many of the commercial hair-care products on the market contain chemicals that can actually do more harm than good. Many shampoos strip hair of moisture or coat it with unnatural chemicals. Instead of alleviating damage, they contribute to it.

Handmade shampoos are an affordable, all-natural alternative. They're easy to whip up (try making a batch with friends—fun!), and they can be adjusted according to hair type and color. They can be used to darken or lighten locks, too.

GENERAL HAIR CARE

There are many factors that influence hair health, including diet, hormones, the hair products we use, and how we care for our hair. Below are some suggestions that can improve the strength, luster, shine, and overall health of your hair.

→ Hair health, like skin health, is determined largely by diet. A balanced diet that includes essential fatty acids and plenty of water is critical for healthy hair. B vitamins and protein are also important for healthy hair. Foods such as whole grains, beans, leafy greens, avocados, nuts, seeds, and lean proteins are wonderful for nurturing healthy locks. A high-nutrient, nourishing herb like the nettle can encourage hair health, thickness, and growth.

→ Hormones play a part in causing your hair to be oily or dry. Today many people suffer from hormone imbalances, which may be natural—part of adolescence, menstruation, pregnancy, or menopause. However, outside factors such as pollution and chemicals can also influence hormone levels. Herbs such as vitex, saw palmetto, and wild yam can help balance hormones. Check out the Additional Resources section on page 138 for books with further information on this subject.

→ If blow-drying is a regular part of your styling regimen, use a cool setting. Hot air can dry out and damage hair.

→ Brushing wet hair can cause it to break and snap. Use a wide-mouth comb on wet hair instead. If your hair is tangled, comb a bit of oil through it to loosen the knots. When you do brush, use a natural-bristle brush. It's easier on the hair than other types of brushes and can help in distributing your hair's natural oils.

→ Head and scalp massages are wonderful for relieving stress and tension and stimulating the scalp. Scalp stimulation increases the flow of blood to the scalp, which brings nourishment to the hair follicles and increases hair growth. Scalp massages are especially great when they're done with a nourishing oil like coconut or jojoba.

What's Your Hair Type?

Curly

Curly hair has a lot of body. Because it dries out easily, it needs to be pampered. If this is your hair type, you should avoid products that are drying and use extra conditioner. And here's a great rule of thumb for girls (and guys!) with curls: Use a comb instead of a brush to get tangles out. Brushes can cause frizz.

Straight

Straight hair is usually lacking in body and bounce. It tends to be limp. As a result, many straight-haired people (including myself) overprocess their locks and use too many products, all in an effort to increase volume. This can cause hair to become dry and damaged. If you've got straight hair, know that it will benefit from brushing. Try giving it a few strokes for added body.

Dry

Dry hair tends to be brittle. It knots and breaks easily. It's often accompanied by split ends and dry scalp, a condition similar to dandruff.

Oily

Oily hair appears stringy and greasy. The condition is usually caused by overly active sebaceous glands in the scalp, which cause it to produce more oil than is necessary for healthy hair.

Damaged

So many people have damaged hair these days! Countless factors cause it—the environment, overuse of products, overdying, over-styling, the list goes on. Damaged hair tends to be dry, with split ends. It can break easily and may be dull rather than shiny.

Dandruff

Dandruff is the excessive shedding of dead skin cells from the scalp. The unsightly cells flake off in clumps. Other symptoms of dandruff include redness, irritation, and itching. Dandruff can be caused and worsened by a number of factors, including allergies to shampoos and other hair products, sweating, environmental conditions, yeasts living in the scalp, and hereditary conditions. It's often mistaken for dry scalp.

Combination

Many people have combination hair. They may have an oily scalp and dry ends. They may also suffer from other hair problems, including dandruff.

HOW TO DO A SCALP MASSAGE

Begin at the forehead. Using both hands, with the fingertips of each just touching at the center of the forehead, lightly apply pressure and release it every few seconds. Slowly move the fingers onto and up the scalp, continuing the pressure-and-release motion. Continue to the base of the scalp at the back of the head. Then move your hands farther apart so that there's about an inch of space between the fingertips of each. Continue the pressure-and-release movement to the front of your scalp. Then move your fingers even farther apart so that there are 2 to 3 inches of space between the fingertips of each. Repeat the action, moving the fingers farther apart each time you reach the front or back of the scalp until the entire scalp has been massaged.

→ Watch out for the wind and the sun. They can dry out your hair. If you plan to be in direct sunlight for more than half an hour, consider wearing a scarf or hat to protect your hair.

→ Avoid overcleansing your hair. Most of us wash our hair way too often—daily or every other day. Because washing the hair strips it of its natural oils, I suggest you try going an extra day or two between shampooings. I wash my hair two or three times a week. Unless your hair is very oily, try washing it in cool water. Hot water can dry out hair and loosen the shafts, which may cause individual strands to fall out.

→ Don't over-style your hair. Most commercial hair products strip hair of moisture. They're also very drying to the scalp. Try to not use styling products more than a couple of times a week.

→ Have your hair trimmed regularly. Getting rid of split ends makes hair appear fuller and healthier. It also helps to prevent breakage.

→ Use the products in this book! You can personalize these shampoos and conditioning treatments so that they suit your hair type. These natural products can help hair gain and retain moisture and nutrients. They can repair damaged, dry, or overprocessed hair and make it stronger, thicker, and shinier.

BASIC HERBAL SHAMPOO

YOU WILL NEED:

- ½ CUP LIQUID CASTILE SOAP
- ½ CUP HERBAL TEA (SEE RECIPE AT RIGHT)
- 1 TABLESPOON GLYCERIN
- 25 TO 40 DROPS ESSENTIAL OIL
- 1 TEASPOON OIL*
- BOWL
- EMPTY SHAMPOO BOTTLE OR PLASTIC SQUEEZE BOTTLE

* (IF YOUR HAIR IS DRY, ADD 1 TO 2 TEASPOONS OF A LIGHT OIL TO THE SHAMPOO. IF YOU HAVE OILY HAIR OR SIMPLY DON'T WANT OIL IN YOUR SHAMPOO, FEEL FREE TO LEAVE IT OUT. JOJOBA, OLIVE, AND GRAPESEED OILS ARE SOME OF MY FAVORITES TO USE IN SHAMPOOS.)

To make the Basic Herbal Shampoo:

(1) Put all of the ingredients in a bowl and stir them well.

(2) Pour the mixture into a plastic squeeze bottle or an empty shampoo bottle.

To use: Shampoo your hair as you normally would, and rinse it well with cool water. Follow with an herbal hair rinse if desired. *Note:* The shampoo will separate and thicken slightly in the bottle, so shake it before you apply it. You can refrigerate it, but make sure you use it before it spoils.

HERBAL TEA RECIPE

YOU WILL NEED:

- ¼ CUP DRIED PLANT MATERIAL
- JAR WITH LID
- 1 CUP DISTILLED WATER
- PLASTIC OR METAL STRAINER OR PIECE OF CHEESECLOTH
- PLASTIC BOWL OR MEASURING CUP

1. Place the plant material in the jar.

2. Bring the water to a boil and pour it into the jar so that the plant material is covered.

3. Put the lid on the jar and let the herbs infuse the water for at least 20 minutes. (I often let mine sit for an hour.)

4. Strain the tea with the strainer or the cheesecloth. You may need to strain it two or three times to get the plant bits out. If some sediment remains after you've strained, don't worry about it.

5. Pour the tea into a plastic bowl or measuring cup. If you have extra tea left over, you can use it to make the Herbal Tea Rinse on page 92.

SHAMPOO TO BRING OUT LOWLIGHTS

To make a shampoo that will darken hair slightly and bring out lowlights, follow the directions for the Basic Herbal Shampoo recipe on page 86. For the herbal-tea portion of the recipe, use 1/8 cup black walnut, 1/8 cup sage, and 1/16 cup marshmallow root. For the essential-oil portion, use rosemary. *Note:* Black walnut tea on its own can stain the skin. When used in this shampoo, it shouldn't be a problem.

SHAMPOO TO BRING OUT HIGHLIGHTS

To make a shampoo that can bring out highlights in your hair, follow the directions for the Basic Herbal Shampoo recipe on page 86. For the herbal-tea portion of the recipe, use 1/8 cup chamomile and 1/8 cup calendula. For the essential-oil portion, use citrus. Add 1 teaspoon of lemon juice.

DANDRUFF SHAMPOO

To make a dandruff-fighting shampoo, follow the directions for the Basic Herbal Shampoo recipe on page 86. For the herbal-tea portion of the recipe, use 1/8 cup rosemary and 1/8 cup sage. For the essential-oil portion, use rosemary, tea tree, and/or myrrh. *Note:* You can also add 1 teaspoon of olive oil to this shampoo, which will help with both dandruff and dryness. Be aware that the sage and rosemary essential oils may slightly darken hair that's light.

SHAMPOO FOR OILY HAIR

If you suffer from oily hair, this is the shampoo for you! To make it, follow the directions for the Basic Herbal Shampoo recipe on page 86. For the herbal-tea portion of the recipe, use 1/4 cup rose. For the essential-oil portion, use clary sage. *Note:* If your hair is both oily and dry, try adding jojoba oil to this shampoo. Jojoba can be helpful in balancing the body's production of oils.

SHAMPOO FOR DRY OR DAMAGED HAIR

This shampoo can restore health to dry, damaged, or brittle hair. To make it, follow the directions for the Basic Herbal Shampoo recipe on page 86. For the herbal-tea portion of the recipe, use 1/8 cup marshmallow root, 1/16 cup borage, and 1/16 cup comfrey. For the essential-oil portion, use lavender and/or peppermint. Add 2 teaspoons of jojoba or sesame oil (keep in mind that sesame has a strong scent that some people find displeasing). *Note:* Marshmallow root can darken hair, especially if it's light or blond. You can substitute peppermint leaf for marshmallow root if you like.

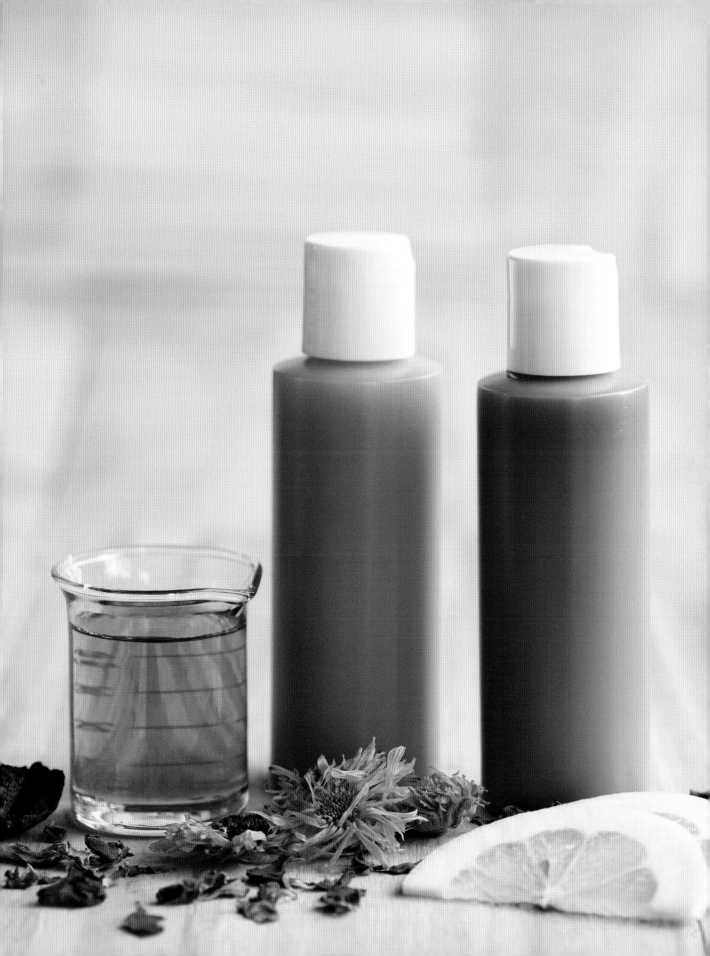

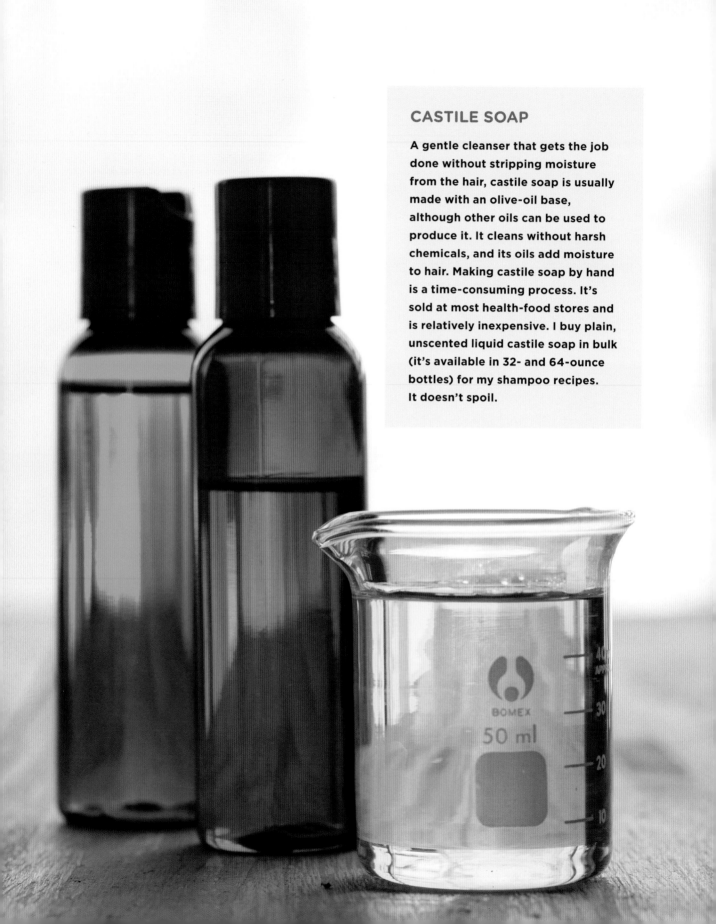

CASTILE SOAP

A gentle cleanser that gets the job done without stripping moisture from the hair, castile soap is usually made with an olive-oil base, although other oils can be used to produce it. It cleans without harsh chemicals, and its oils add moisture to hair. Making castile soap by hand is a time-consuming process. It's sold at most health-food stores and is relatively inexpensive. I buy plain, unscented liquid castile soap in bulk (it's available in 32- and 64-ounce bottles) for my shampoo recipes. It doesn't spoil.

HAIR OILS FOR CONDITIONING

Hair is one of the few physical characteristics that we can easily alter. I won't lie—I love to dye mine. This year, I've gone from blond to raven black. I generally use natural products like henna to color my hair, but for dramatic changes, I go to a salon. As a result, my hair tends to be dry and damaged. It's also thin and prone to split ends. Pampering it is important, so I give it an extra bit of love with a replenishing hot-oil treatment.

All-natural hot-oil treatments are incredibly easy to put together. My favorite recipe follows.

HOT-OIL TREATMENT FOR DRY, DAMAGED HAIR

YOU WILL NEED:

- 2 TABLESPOONS COCONUT OIL
- 2 TABLESPOONS JOJOBA OIL
- 2 TABLESPOONS ARGON OIL
- 5 DROPS ESSENTIAL OIL OF YOUR CHOICE (OPTIONAL)
- POT OR SAUCEPAN
- GLASS MEASURING CUP
- SMALL WIDE-MOUTHED CONTAINER WITH LID

(1) Create a simple double boiler for warming the coconut oil. Put about two inches of water in the pot and warm it over low heat. Put the coconut oil in the measuring cup, and place the cup in the pot. Once the coconut oil has melted, take the cup out of the pot.

(2) Add the jojoba and argon oils to the cup of melted coconut oil.

(3) Add the essential oil (if desired) and stir.

(4) Pour the oil into the container.

To use: The oil will melt in your hands as you spread it through your hair. (When I apply it to my own hair, I concentrate on the tips.) After the oil has been thoroughly distributed through your hair, put on a plastic shower cap. (In addition to the shower cap, I usually wrap a towel around my head to generate some heat, which can help the oil penetrate my hair. Sitting in the sun helps the oil work, too.) After 20 to 30 minutes, wash your hair as you normally would.

Depending on the length and thickness of your hair, the recipe makes about 3 to 6 treatments. If you have dry, damaged hair, try using the treatment weekly. If your hair isn't all that damaged or is on the oily side, use it once a month or so.

HAIR OIL FOR DANDRUFF

This oil is great if your hair needs conditioning and you suffer from dandruff. Texture-wise, it's a liquid rather than a semi-solid.

YOU WILL NEED:

- 4 TABLESPOONS OLIVE OIL
- 1 TABLESPOON ARGON OIL
- 1 TABLESPOON JOJOBA OIL
- 10 DROPS CLARY SAGE ESSENTIAL OIL
- SMALL BOWL
- SMALL WIDE-MOUTHED CONTAINER WITH LID

(1) Combine the olive, argon, and jojoba oils in the bowl.

(2) Add the essential oil and stir.

(3) Transfer the oil to the container.

To use: Follow the directions for the Hot-Oil Treatment for Dry, Damaged Hair (at left). Depending on the length and thickness of your hair, the recipe makes about 3 to 6 treatments.

OIL FOR COMBINATION HAIR

This is a great recipe for those who have combination hair (oily scalp and dry tips) or oily hair. It helps balance the body's production of oil.

YOU WILL NEED:

- 6 TABLESPOONS JOJOBA OIL
- 10 DROPS CLARY SAGE ESSENTIAL OIL
- SMALL BOWL
- SMALL WIDE-MOUTHED CONTAINER WITH A LID FOR STORING

(1) Put the jojoba oil and the clary sage essential oil in a small bowl, and stir.

(2) Transfer the mixture to the container.

To use: Follow the directions for using the Hot-Oil Treatment for Dry, Damaged Hair on page 91.

HERBAL TEA RINSES

Easy to make and oh-so-nourishing, herbal hair rinses can be used right after washing or in between shampoos. They deliver vitamins and minerals to the hair and can bring out subtle tints and color. Because tea rinses don't keep well, I make one treatment at a time and use it immediately.

BASIC HERBAL TEA RINSE

YOU WILL NEED:

- ¼ CUP DRIED PLANT MATERIAL
- JAR WITH LID
- 1 CUP WATER
- POT OR SAUCEPAN
- PLASTIC OR METAL STRAINER OR PIECE OF CHEESECLOTH
- PLASTIC BOWL OR MEASURING CUP

(1) Place the plant material in the jar.

(2) Put the water in the pot, boil it, and then pour it into the jar so that it covers the plant material thoroughly.

(3) Put the lid on the jar, and let the plant material infuse the water for at least 20 minutes. (I often let mine sit for an hour.)

(4) Strain the tea with the strainer or the cheesecloth. You may need to strain it two or three times to get the plant bits out. If some sediment remains after you've strained, don't worry about it.

(5) Pour the tea into a plastic bowl or measuring cup.

To use: Shampoo and rinse your hair as you normally do. Then pour the rinse over your hair and work it through to the tips. I use a plastic measuring cup when I apply the rinse because

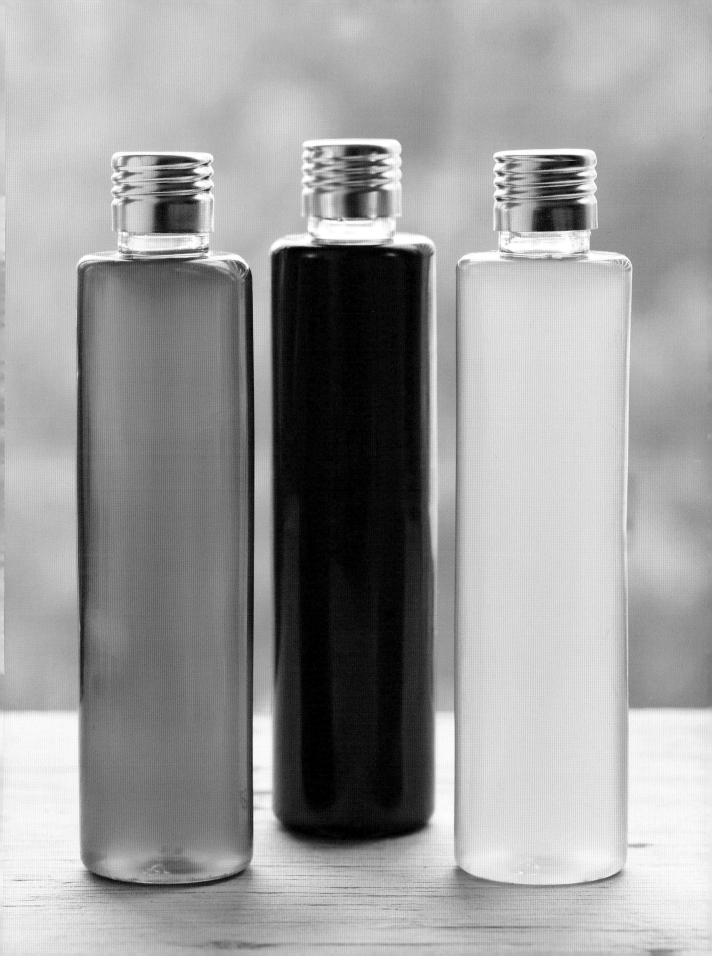

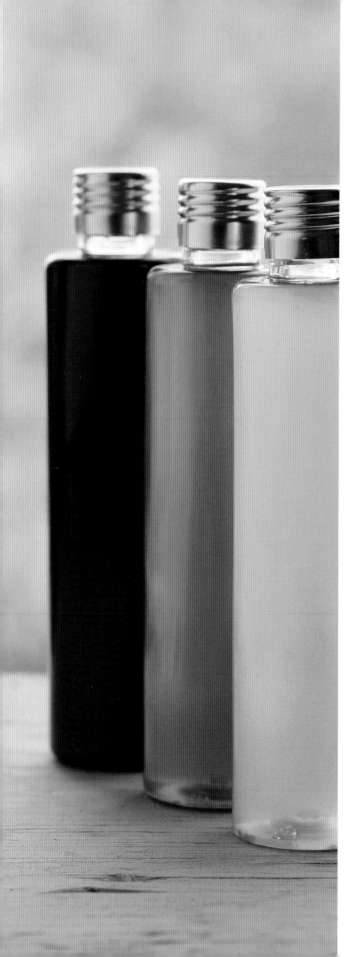

the spout makes it easy to pour. You don't need to rinse your hair with water after you apply the treatment, although you can if you want to.

NETTLE-COMFREY SUPER HAIR-NOURISHER

To make this treatment, add ⅛ cup dried nettles and ⅛ cup comfrey to the Basic Herbal Tea Rinse Recipe on page 92, and follow the directions as listed.

HAIR RINSE FOR HIGHLIGHTS

To make this treatment, add ⅛ cup chamomile and ⅛ cup calendula to the Basic Herbal Tea Rinse Recipe on page 92, and follow the directions as listed.

HAIR RINSE FOR LOWLIGHTS

To make this treatment, add ¼ cup black walnut hull to the Basic Herbal Tea Rinse Recipe on page 92, and follow the directions as listed. *Note:* Black walnut hulls can stain the skin.

SALT HAIR VOLUMIZER

My hair tends to be limp and thin looking—except when I'm at the beach. I wanted to recreate the windswept texture and fullness of beach hair at home, so I created this saltwater volumizer. Similar to the products you see in salons, this all-natural spray costs much less and is easy to make.

A great body-booster that also helps curls hold, this spray is nourishing thanks to the aloe and the oil in the recipe, and the salt makes it cleansing. Try personalizing it by using an oil and an essential oil that suit your hair type.

YOU WILL NEED:

- 1 CUP WATER
- POT OR SAUCEPAN
- 3 TABLESPOONS SALT (I USUALLY USE SEA SALT. EPSOM SALT ALSO WORKS WELL.)
- 1 TEASPOON ALOE VERA GEL
- 1 TEASPOON JOJOBA OIL
- 1 TEASPOON ALCOHOL (AS A PRESERVATIVE)
- SPRAY BOTTLE
- 10 DROPS ESSENTIAL OIL OF YOUR CHOICE (CITRUS OILS ARE GOOD FOR THIS RECIPE.)

1 Heat the water in the pot or saucepan, but don't let it boil.

2 Add the salt. Stir until it's dissolved.

3 Remove the mixture from the heat. Add the aloe vera gel, the jojoba oil, and the alcohol, and stir.

4 Transfer the volumizer to the spray bottle, and add the essential oils.

To use: Shake the volumizer before you use it to distribute the oils. You can apply it to wet or dry hair.

LEMON-COCONUT HAIR LIGHTENER

When I was a child, my mom used a spray-on hair product called Sun-In® during the summer. She'd spray it on her hair before spending time in the sun, and it would brighten her tresses and bring out highlights. In high school, my sister, Sarah, learned that using lemon and chamomile could have the same result on the hair.

Unlike many of the hair-lightening products on the market today, mine is highly nourishing.

YOU WILL NEED:

- 1 CUP CHAMOMILE TEA
- SMALL BOWL
- 1 TEASPOON COCONUT OIL
- ¼ CUP LEMON JUICE
- 1 TEASPOON ALCOHOL
- 1 TEASPOON ALOE VERA GEL
- LEMON OR CHAMOMILE ESSENTIAL OIL (OPTIONAL)
- SPRAY BOTTLE

1 To make the chamomile tea, follow the steps in the Herbal Tea Recipe on page 87. Use ¼ cup dried chamomile.

2 After the tea has been strained, but while it's still warm, transfer it to a small bowl and add the coconut oil. Stir until the coconut oil has melted, and then allow the mixture to cool to room temperature.

3 Add the lemon juice, the alcohol, and the aloe vera gel, and stir.

4 Add the lemon or chamomile essential oil if desired, and transfer the mixture to the spray bottle.

To use: Spray the lightener on your locks before going outside. The sun will bring out natural highlights in your hair. Make sure you store the lightener in the fridge—it won't keep well otherwise.

BATH

Is there anything more relaxing—or magical—than an herbal bath? A nice soak sweetened with natural bath salts can calm and quiet the mind, encourage deep sleep, and provide comfort after a stressful day. Depending on the herbs used and the temperature of the water, a bath can stimulate and uplift or relax and soothe. It can decongest the chest and the head, reduce a fever, or ease a migraine.

Herbal baths have a long history and have been used for generations to successfully treat stress, respiratory ailments, achy muscles, and fevers. Baths were once one of the main methods practitioners used to deliver herbal medicine. Hot water opens pores and makes it easy for the skin to absorb the healing properties of herbs. Hand and foot baths are also effective. Never underestimate the power of a good soak!

BATH SALTS

Bath salts soften water while adding valuable minerals to it. And, of course, they cleanse the skin. Simple to assemble, they make great giveaways or party favors—no girl can resist a fresh batch of bath salts! (For suggestions on fun, creative ways to package your salts and other products, see the Packaging Ideas section beginning on page 123.) Displayed on a shelf, salts can add sparkle to your bathroom. Salts come in different colors, so you can change up the shades you use to create pretty, decorative effects.

BASIC BATH SALT

YOU WILL NEED:

- 2 CUPS SALT
- 1 CUP DRIED HERB MIXTURE OF YOUR CHOICE
- ½ CUP CLAY (OPTIONAL)
- ½ CUP BORAX (OPTIONAL)
- LARGE BOWL
- 25 DROPS ESSENTIAL OIL OF YOUR CHOICE
- SEVERAL GLASS JARS WITH LIDS OR PLASTIC BAGS

(1) In a large bowl, mix all of the ingredients together except for the essential oils. Stir thoroughly.

(2) Sprinkle the essential oils over the mixture and then stir them in. Mix the ingredients well.

(3) Pour the salt into the glass jars or plastic bags and seal.

WHY AM I ADDING BORAX TO MY BATH SALTS?!

Borax is a naturally occurring mineral composed of sodium, boron, oxygen, and water. Commonly used as an alkaline water softener and cleansing agent, it's useful in mineral-bath blends. Some recipes out there call for more borax than I use in my bath blends, so feel free to experiment with the amount until you find what works best. (I've seen recipes that call for twice as much borax as salt!) Keep in mind that borax can cause bath salts to clump if they get wet or aren't sealed properly. So if your water is already soft or you simply don't like the effects of borax, you can omit it altogether.

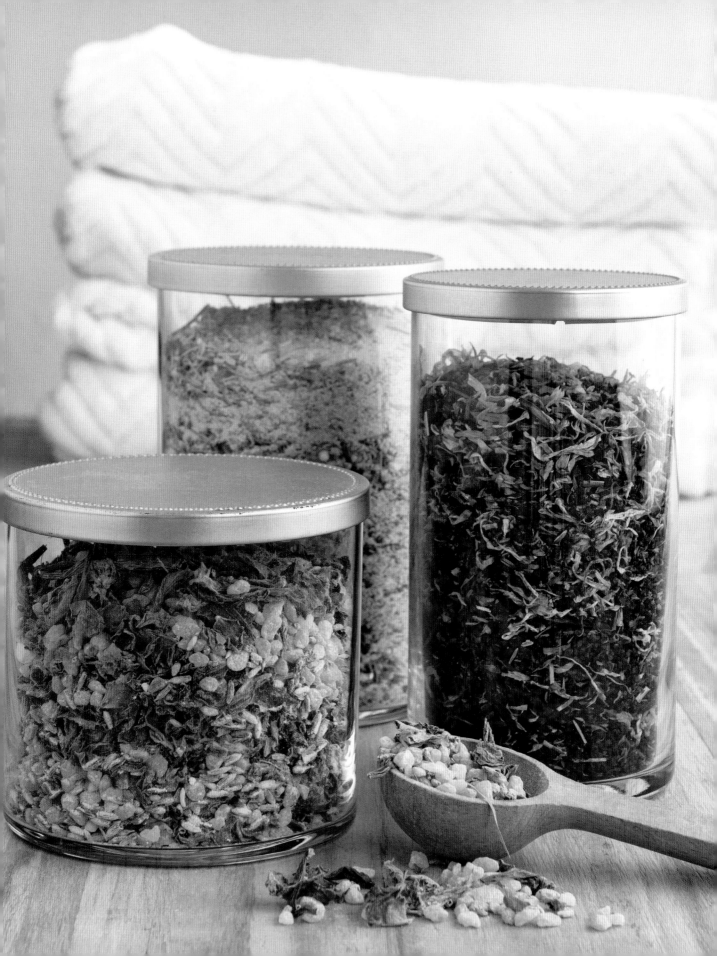

BLACK MAGIC BATH SALT

To make this salt, follow the directions for the Basic Bath Salt recipe (page 96), and use black salt. For the herb-mixture portion of the recipe, use calendula, St. John's wort, and borage. Add red clay and bergamot essential oil.

PINK LOVE BATH SALT

To make this salt, follow the directions for the Basic Bath Salt recipe (page 96), and use pink salt. For the herb-mixture portion of the recipe, use rose, lavender, and borage. Add kaolin clay and ylang ylang essential oil.

HERBAL SEA BATH SALT

To make this salt, follow the directions for the Basic Bath Salt recipe (page 96), and use sea salt. For the herb-mixture portion of the recipe, use rosemary, sage, and chamomile. Add kaolin clay and lavender essential oil.

EPSOM SALT SORE-MUSCLE SOAK

To make this salt, follow the directions for the Basic Bath Salt recipe (page 96), and use Epsom salt. For the herb-mixture portion of the recipe, use arnica and sage. Add kaolin clay and rosemary essential oil.

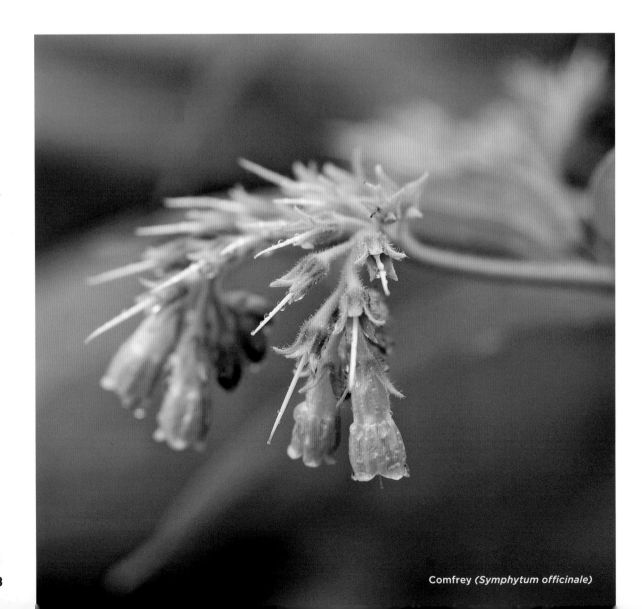

Comfrey (Symphytum officinale)

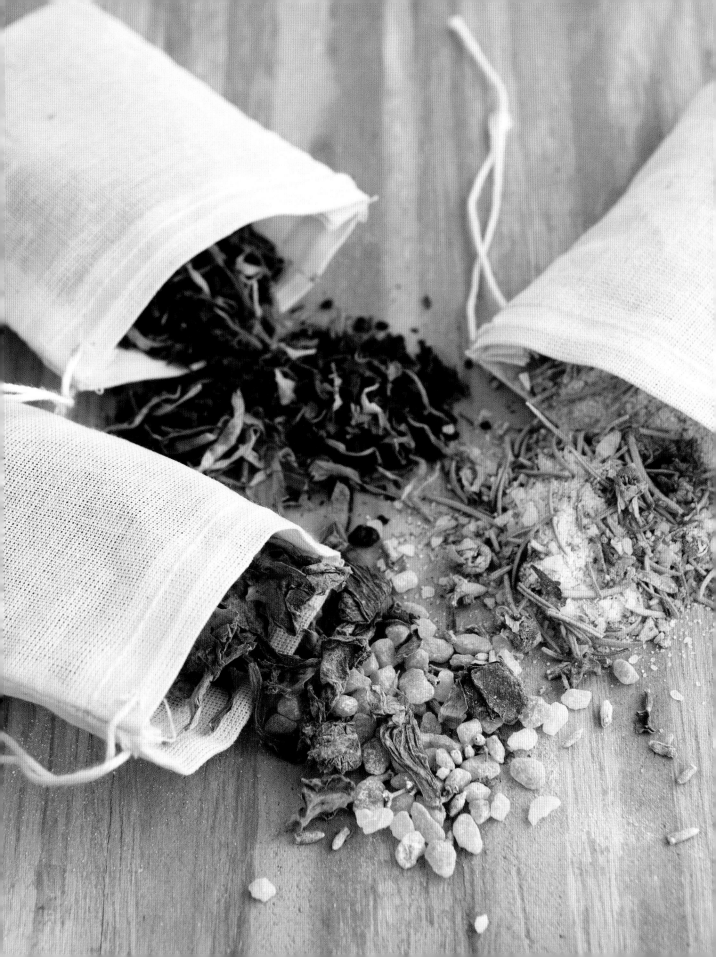

BATH SOAKS

Bath soaks are like bathing in a wonderful, healing herbal tea! They're incredibly easy to make using one of the methods below.

→ Add herbs directly to hot bath water. I love this method, especially when I'm using flowers like borage or rose. However, the process can be messy, and you'll want to clean the tub when you're done.

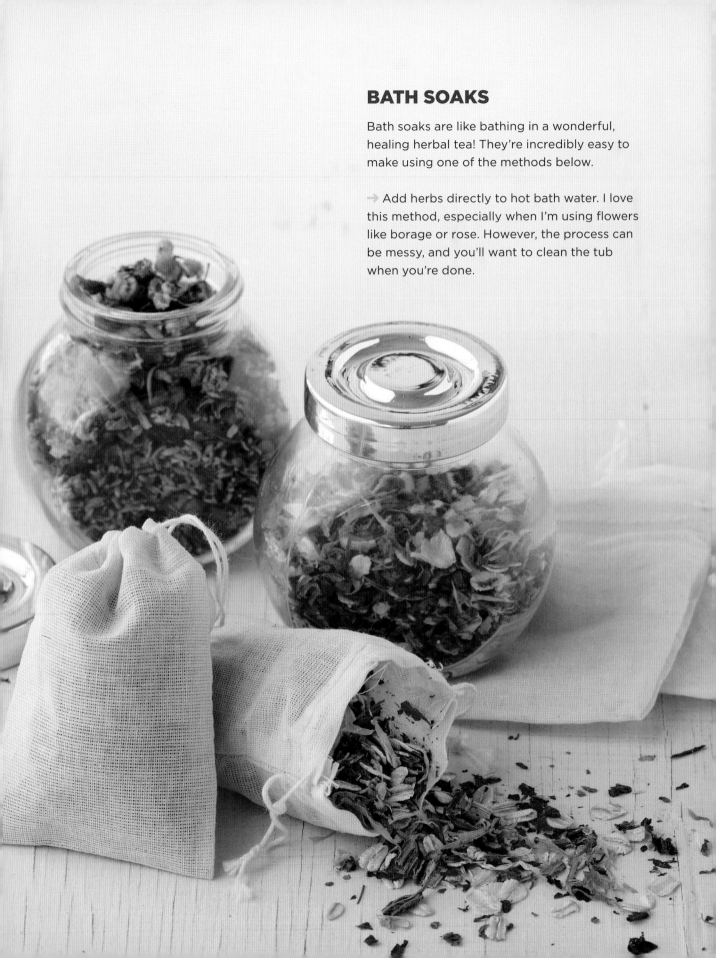

→ Put the herbs in a cloth "tea bag," and submerge it in your bath water. This method works very well and isn't messy. You can purchase muslin drawstring bags for this purpose, or make your own. A clean sock will also do the trick. Just place the herb-filled bag in the tub with you while you soak, or use it as a washcloth.

→ Use bath soaks to make a strong tea that you add to your bath water. Put 1 cup of the herbs of your choice in a pint jar, fill the jar with boiling water, and cover it. Let the herbs steep in the water for at least 20 minutes, and then strain them with a strainer or a piece of cheesecloth. Pour the resulting tea into your bath.

To Make Bath Soaks

Combine equal amounts of the dried herbs listed in each recipe in a jar. Then use one of the methods listed above to add them to your bath.

SUPER SKIN NOURISHER

Oatmeal, nettles, comfrey, calendula, chickweed

BATH SOAK FOR RASHES, BUG BITES, OR DRY, ITCHY SKIN

Great for kids! Calendula, oats, and chickweed

SLEEPY

Wonderful for relaxing babies, kids, and adults. Lavender, chamomile, roses, borage

WAKE UP

Perfect if you need a mental or physical pick-me-up. Rosemary, sage, peppermint

AMANDA'S SUGAR-SCRUB

This recipe was contributed by my sister. It has a yummy, rich smell and is wonderful for exfoliating rough heels and elbows. A great scrub for the entire body that cleanses and moisturizes, it'll clear away dead skin cells and leave you feeling polished.

YOU WILL NEED:

- 2 CUPS BROWN SUGAR
- 2 CUPS WHITE SUGAR
- LARGE BOWL
- 1 TABLESPOON + 1 TEASPOON POWDERED CINNAMON
- 1 TABLESPOON + 1 TEASPOON POWDERED GINGER
- 1 TABLESPOON + 1 TEASPOON POWDERED NUTMEG
- 1 TABLESPOON + 1 TEASPOON POWDERED CARDAMOM
- 1½ CUPS OIL (PREFERABLY A NUT OIL LIKE ALMOND OR HAZELNUT. SOY IS ALSO AN OPTION.)
- 40 DROPS ESSENTIAL OIL OF ONE OR COMBINATION OF CINNAMON, GINGER, NUTMEG, AND CARDAMOM
- SEVERAL JARS WITH LIDS

(1) Combine the brown sugar, the white sugar, and the powdered spices in a bowl, and mix them well with your hands or a wooden spoon.

(2) Add the oil and the essential oil. Stir the ingredients until they're thoroughly combined and the mixture resembles damp sand.

(3) Transfer the scrub to the jars, and store.

To use: Massage the scrub into the skin, focusing on rough, dry areas. Rinse with warm water.

FACE

Skin: It's the human body's largest organ. It plays a critical part in human health by protecting the body from physical, biological, and chemical threats. It supplies us with a sense of touch, and helps the body maintain its proper temperature and moisture levels through sweating. It also stores and metabolizes fat, secretes an oil called sebum, and helps our bodies eliminate unwanted materials and toxins.

The face is one of the most sensitive and problematic regions of the skin, and it requires special care. Many of the commercial products available today are overdrying and do more harm than good to this vulnerable area. Herbal facial products are a wonderful, easy-to-make alternative.

GENERAL SKIN CARE

While the recipes in this book can help improve skin appearance and health, you should remember that beauty comes from the inside out. What we put in our bodies is more important than the products we use on our skin.

→ Make sure you eat a healthy, well-balanced diet that includes lots of vitamins and minerals. Drink plenty of water. If your body is dehydrated, then your skin will be, too.

→ Keep your liver healthy. It's the main place where the body processes toxins. If your liver isn't functioning properly, your skin will start processing toxins, which can cause breakouts, oily or dry skin, and dermatological problems like eczema. Our bodies are forced to process many potentially harmful chemicals and substances, and this taxes an already hard-working liver. Foods such as beets, leafy greens, and avocados, as well as herbs like dandelion root, burdock root, and milk-thistle seeds support liver health. Visit the Additional

Resources section on page 138 for a list of books that cover liver health, nutrition, and the internal use of herbs.

→ Eliminating or reducing your toxin intake can boost liver and skin health. Cutting back on alcohol, sugar, caffeine, and cigarettes will make a huge difference in how you look and feel. Here's a personal example: I never had a problem with acne until I was in college and began smoking cigarettes. My skin broke out, and I had a hunch the flare-ups were caused by my smoking habit (and probably the stress of studying). Once I quit, my skin cleared up. So I encourage you to look at your habits, both bad and good, and to take note of patterns and changes in your skin and in your overall health.

→ A key part of maintaining overall health and good skin, exercise helps to bring extra blood and oxygen to the skin. The blood then carries away debris and waste, thereby cleaning the skin cells. Exercise decreases stress and can be a powerful mood-booster. It can also help with skin conditions that are exacerbated by stress, including acne, eczema, and psoriasis.

DRY BRUSHING

A great way to exfoliate, dry brushing is best done before a bath or shower, as it opens up the pores. Try it with a loofah or a natural-bristle body brush. It can stimulate blood flow, remove dead skin cells, and help rid the body of toxins. Dry brushing may also help smooth spots of cellulite. It will definitely leave your skin with a healthy, rosy glow! It can be done up to twice a day. Your skin should feel tingly and invigorated afterward—not irritated. Note: Always dry brush toward your heart.

→ Sleep is just as important as exercise. If your body is tired, your skin will show it. Lack of sleep makes blood vessels dilate, which can lead to a blotchy complexion and dark under-eye circles. Sleep is the time your body and your skin cells use to repair themselves. A good night's sleep can be a huge boost to overall skin health.

→ Stress, as we all know, is hard on the body. It can do damage internally and externally. Most of us are under some form of continual stress and live in "fight-or-flight" mode. Finding healthy ways to relieve stress—through massage, exercise, or relaxing baths—can do wonders for the body.

→ Regular exfoliation of the skin is important, as it removes dead cells and makes way for healthy new ones. Exfoliating through dry-skin brushing or with one of the cleansers featured in this book also brings extra blood to the skin, which (like exercise) helps to deliver oxygen and get rid of toxins.

→ Here comes the sun! Get a little sunlight on bare skin (with no sunscreen) for 20 to 60 minutes a day, depending on your skin tone and coloring (20 minutes for light and up to 60 for dark skin). This is best done when the sun is at its least potent (before 10 a.m. or after 4 p.m.). The sun gives the body vitamin D, which helps rid it of cancer-causing free radicals. It helps the skin retain moisture and boosts the body's immune system, which can help with skin problems such as acne. Vitamin D also assists with cell proliferation, which encourages healthy skin-cell growth. But always remember that less is more when it comes to the sun. Overexposure can do more harm than good to your skin.

→ Try the recipes in this book! When you use products that have been customized to suit your needs (and made with love and care!), you'll be amazed at the improvement in your skin.

BASIC SKIN TYPES

Normal-to-balanced skin is the ideal type. It's neither oily nor dry, which means that it's performing all the duties of healthy skin and functioning as it should. It looks radiant and supple.

Oily skin is characterized by overactive sebaceous glands and large, visible pores. It tends to be greasy and can be accompanied by acne. Oily skin isn't usually sensitive.

Dry skin lacks natural oil and moisture. In appearance, it can be dry, scaly, and wrinkled, with small pores. Dry skin is easily irritated. Superficially dry skin can be caused by the environment. The wind, the sun, and various pollutants can make any skin type appear dry, as can skin conditions such as eczema, psoriasis, and dermatitis.

Combination skin is a mix of the above types, each of which can occur on a different part of the face. The forehead, nose, and chin may be oily or balanced, while the cheeks and the area around the eyes may be dry. Most people have this type of skin.

Sensitive skin is easily irritated by everything from the environment to body-care products and cosmetics. It may itch or burn and be red or rashy in appearance. It's also prone to broken capillaries and sunburn.

CLAY MASKS

Easy to make and fun to try (the best part is waiting for the clay to dry and looking like a monster in the meantime)! Clay draws out dirt and toxins, tightens pores, and leaves the skin looking clear, clean, and rosy. Clay can be drying, though, so don't apply a mask more than once a week. I follow mine with a moisturizer (see Rosemary Gladstar's Perfect Cream on page 116).

BASIC CLAY MASK

YOU WILL NEED:

- 1 CUP CLAY
- 2 TABLESPOONS GROUND HERBS
- BOWL
- WIDE-MOUTHED CONTAINER

(1) Mix the clay and the herbs together in a bowl. Stir them thoroughly.

(2) Pour the mixture into the container.

To use: This recipe makes about 8 ounces of dry clay mask. A little goes a long way. Add a small amount of water to 1 to 2 tablespoons of clay. Mix the two together in the palm of your hand (or in a small bowl) with your fingers. Then spread the clay over your face in a circular motion using your fingers. Allow the mask to dry. You'll feel it tightening up your skin. After it has dried, rinse it off thoroughly with warm water or remove it with a washcloth.

Depending on the type of clay you use, you can alter the appearance and the effects of the mask.

OILY SKIN

To make a mask for oily skin, follow the directions for the Basic Clay Mask recipe above and use red clay, lavender, and rosemary.

DRY SKIN

To make a mask for dry skin, follow the directions for the Basic Clay Mask recipe (at left) and use kaolin clay, borage, and calendula.

ACNE-PRONE SKIN

To make a mask for acne-prone skin, follow the directions for the Basic Clay Mask recipe (at left) and use red clay, sage, and chamomile.

FOR COMBINATION SKIN

To make a mask for combination skin, follow the instructions for the Basic Clay Mask recipe (at left) and use bentonite or green clay, lavender, and rose.

GUEST RECIPE:
AMY'S HERBAL-HONEY FACIAL MASK

This recipe was contributed by my friend and former teacher, Amy.

Combining the detoxifying properties of honey and neem, this mask purifies the skin while nourishing it with fenugreek, violet, rose, and oats. Honey removes toxins and bacteria while healing abrasions and wounds. It's safe enough for delicate or dry skin, but strong enough to cleanse effectively and fight acne. Don't forget: Give thanks to the bees with every use!

YOU WILL NEED:

- ½ TEASPOON EACH OF THE FOLLOWING POWDERED HERBS: FENUGREEK, GOTU KOLA, NEEM, OATS, ROSE PETALS, AND VIOLET LEAF (YOU CAN USE CUT AND SIFTED HERBS, BUT POWDER MAKES FOR A SMOOTHER APPLICATION TO THE FACE.)
- 2 OUNCES LOCAL HONEY
- LARGE BOWL
- JAR WITH LID
- 10 DROPS SANDALWOOD OR ROSE ESSENTIAL OIL

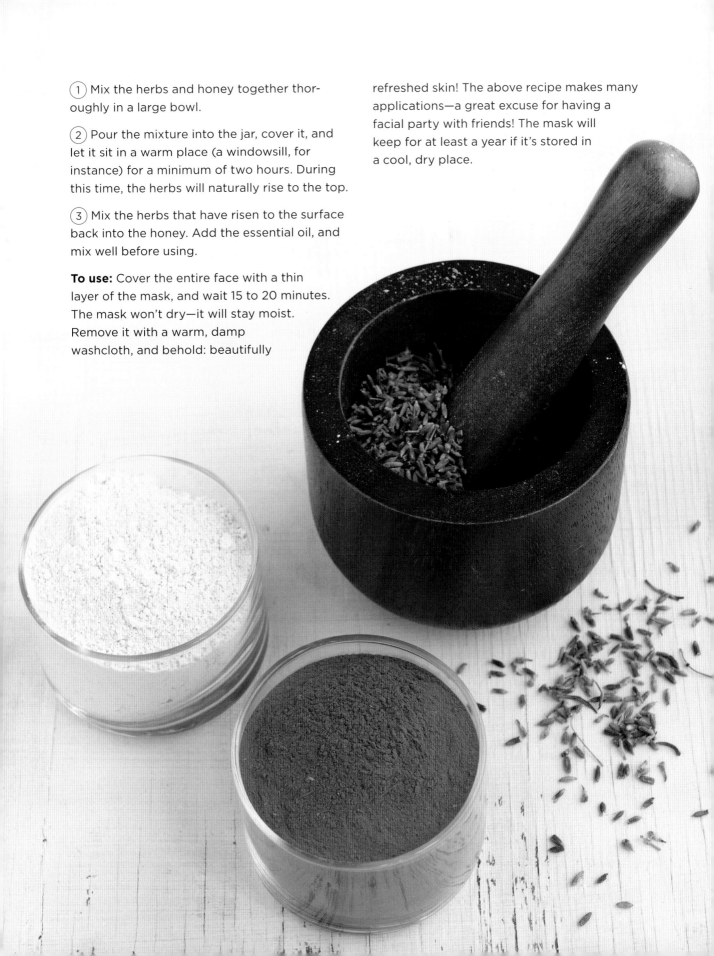

(1) Mix the herbs and honey together thoroughly in a large bowl.

(2) Pour the mixture into the jar, cover it, and let it sit in a warm place (a windowsill, for instance) for a minimum of two hours. During this time, the herbs will naturally rise to the top.

(3) Mix the herbs that have risen to the surface back into the honey. Add the essential oil, and mix well before using.

To use: Cover the entire face with a thin layer of the mask, and wait 15 to 20 minutes. The mask won't dry—it will stay moist. Remove it with a warm, damp washcloth, and behold: beautifully refreshed skin! The above recipe makes many applications—a great excuse for having a facial party with friends! The mask will keep for at least a year if it's stored in a cool, dry place.

ROSEMARY GLADSTAR'S MIRACLE GRAINS

The wonderful herbalist, Rosemary Gladstar, generously provided two recipes for this book, as well as insight and tips for achieving the best results. Here's what she has to say.

I love washing my face with these Miracle Grains. When you see how wonderfully radiant and soft your face is after using them, you'll find it hard to go back to your old cleanser.

The perfect substitute for soap, cleansing grains are mild, nourishing, suitable for all skin types, and safe enough for daily use. Many commercial cleansing grains are too harsh—they feel like sandpaper on the skin. Teenagers with breakouts often use those rough cleansers, thinking they'll scrub the acne away. Not so! Skin—especially blemished skin—should be treated gently. Harsh cleansers will only further irritate an already-inflamed condition.

The light grains in this recipe are perfect for blemished skin. They cleanse gently, redistribute excess oil, remove dead cells, and improve circulation. You can add a number of different items (seaweed, vitamins A and E, and other combinations of herbs) to my basic recipe. Be creative! Try designing a wonderful formula for yourself—one that's truly unique and just right for your skin type. You may want to add a few drops of essential oils such as lavender, rose, or lemon balm to enhance the scent and the effect of the grains. Make sure the oils are pure and not synthetic; synthetic oils can burn and irritate the skin.

YOU WILL NEED:

- 2 CUPS KAOLIN CLAY
- 1 CUP FINELY GROUND OATS
- ¼ CUP FINELY GROUND ALMONDS
- ⅛ CUP FINELY GROUND LAVENDER
- ⅛ CUP POPPY SEEDS OR FINELY GROUND BLUE CORN (OPTIONAL)
- ⅛ CUP FINELY GROUND ROSES
- LARGE BOWL
- GLASS CONTAINER OR SPICE JAR WITH SHAKER TOP

Combine all of the ingredients in a large bowl, and mix them well. Then transfer the mixture to a glass container or spice jar with a shaker top.

To use: Dispense 1 to 2 teaspoons of the cleansing grains into very wet hands, and create a creamy paste by rubbing the palms together. Apply to the face in circular motions, avoiding the eye area. Massage gently for one minute, then rinse thoroughly.

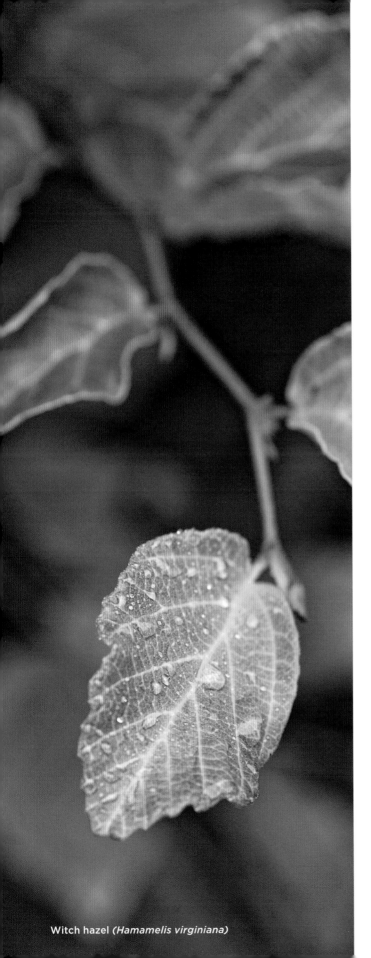

TONERS AND ASTRINGENTS

Simple to make and wonderfully refreshing for the complexion, toners and astringents are a great way to clean the skin and tighten pores.

BASIC WITCH HAZEL ASTRINGENT

This simple recipe can be put together using ready-made witch hazel extract, which is widely available and relatively inexpensive. (If you prefer, you can make your own witch hazel extract by following the instructions for making a tincture on page 74.) You don't have to use an essential oil in this recipe, but it can help maximize the healing ability of the astringent. If you do use an essential oil, choose one that has a scent you like and that complements your skin type. Lavender and peppermint are some of my favorites.

YOU WILL NEED:

- ½ CUP WITCH HAZEL EXTRACT
- ½ CUP DISTILLED WATER
- SMALL BOWL
- 25 TO 30 DROPS ESSENTIAL OIL (OPTIONAL)
- SPRAY BOTTLE OR LIDDED CONTAINER

(1) Put the water and the witch-hazel extract in the bowl, and mix them together.

(2) Add the essential oil if desired, and transfer the astringent to a spray bottle or lidded container.

To use: Shake the astringent before you apply it. Spray it on the face after cleansing or use it as a refreshing spritzer during the day. You can also apply it with a cotton ball.

Witch hazel (*Hamamelis virginiana*)

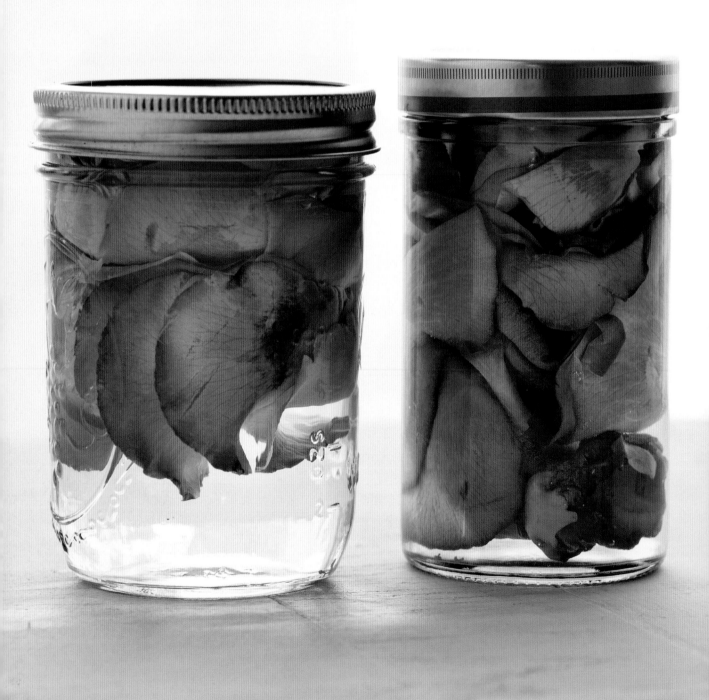

TOYIA'S VANILLA-ROSE TONER

The roses used in this fragrant, refreshing toner are more astringing than witch hazel and compatible with any skin type. If possible, you should use organic roses in this recipe, as conventionally grown roses are often sprayed with chemicals, and you don't want chemicals to be infused in your toner.

This recipe was contributed by my first herb teacher, Toyia.

YOU WILL NEED:

- CLEAN JAR WITH LID
- FRESH ROSE PETALS (PREFERABLY ORGANIC)
- 1 VANILLA BEAN
- WITCH HAZEL EXTRACT
- SPRAY BOTTLE OR SMALL LIDDED CONTAINER

1. Put the rose petals in the jar until it's nearly full (or take the jar with you when you gather the petals, and place them in it).

2. Add the vanilla bean to the jar, and then fill the jar with the witch hazel extract, making sure that all of the plant matter is submerged.

3. Close the jar and let the mixture infuse for 2 to 6 weeks away from direct sunlight. Shake the jar daily.

4. Strain your lovely toner and enjoy!

To use: After cleansing, apply the toner to your face with a cotton ball, or spritz it on the skin lightly. Follow with your favorite moisturizer. The toner will keep longer if it's stored in a cool place, but it doesn't need to be refrigerated.

TONER FOR ACNE

This antimicrobial toner is helpful for treating acne with a bacterial component.

YOU WILL NEED:

- ½ CUP LEMON BALM OR SAGE ALCOHOL EXTRACT (FOLLOW THE DIRECTIONS FOR MAKING A TINCTURE ON PAGE 74)
- ½ CUP DISTILLED WATER
- 1 TEASPOON ALOE VERA GEL
- SMALL BOWL
- 10 DROPS THYME ESSENTIAL OIL
- 10 DROPS MYRRH ESSENTIAL OIL
- 10 DROPS TEA TREE ESSENTIAL OIL
- SPRAY BOTTLE OR SMALL LIDDED CONTAINER

1. Put the water, the lemon balm extract, and the aloe vera gel in the bowl, and stir well.

2. Add the essential oils, and then transfer the toner to a spray bottle or small lidded container.

To use: Shake the toner before you use it. Spray it on the face after cleansing, or use it as a refreshing spritzer during the day. You can also apply it with a cotton ball.

BAY RUM

A classic scent in aftershaves and soaps, bay rum has long been favored by men as a fragrance. Legend has it that during the 1500s, sailors in the West Indies rubbed themselves down with the sweet-smelling leaves of the bay tree to camouflage the unappealing body odors that developed during months spent at sea. The steeping of bay leaves in rum to extract their essential oils for use in cologne is a practice that's been going on for centuries.

My own recipe uses kitchen bay leaves and rum, although you can use any type of alcohol. You probably have the rest of the ingredients in your kitchen right now. A wonderful gift for the men in your life, Bay Rum Aftershave firms and tightens pores and helps fight acne.

- ½ CUP BAY LEAVES
- CLEAN JAR WITH LID
- 7 TO 9 WHOLE CLOVES
- 1 CINNAMON STICK
- ¾ CUP RUM (OR OTHER ALCOHOL)
- ¼ CUP DISTILLED WATER

(1) Place the bay leaves and the other herbs in a jar.

(2) Pour in rum or another alcohol. It should cover the herbs by 1 to 3 inches.

(3) Set the jar in a warm spot out of direct light. Let sit for 4 weeks, shaking occasionally.

(4) Strain the liquid well and rebottle.

BAY RUM AFTERSHAVE AND TONER

YOU WILL NEED:

- ½ CUP BAY RUM (SEE RECIPE TO THE LEFT)
- ½ CUP DISTILLED WATER
- 1 TEASPOON ALOE VERA GEL
- SMALL BOWL
- 20 TO 30 DROPS ESSENTIAL OIL (BAY, CLOVE, LAVENDER, ROSEMARY, OR AN OIL WITH A PINEY SCENT)
- BOTTLE OR CONTAINER WITH LID

(1) Put the water, the Bay Rum, and the aloe vera in the bowl, and mix them well.

(2) Add the essential oils, and stir. Transfer the mixture to a bottle or lidded container.

To use: Shake the toner before you use it. Apply it to the face after cleansing, or use it as a refreshing spritzer after shaving. You can also apply it with a cotton ball.

OTHER PRODUCTS FOR MEN

While I think of my recipes as being gender neutral, if I make products for men, I tweak the formulas a bit. As a first step, I consider the skin and hair type of the guy who'll be using the product. I also think about whether or not we need to address special issues like acne or dryness. Then I consider my scent palette. I don't use floral scents like rose or ylang ylang in my recipes for men. Instead, I opt for earthy, woodsy smells like myrrh, rosemary, cedar, and pine, which make the products feel more masculine. In place of flowers, I use leafy plant matter—rosemary, sage, or peppermint. Of course, all of this depends on the person who'll be using the product. Some men out there love flowers and feminine-scented items!

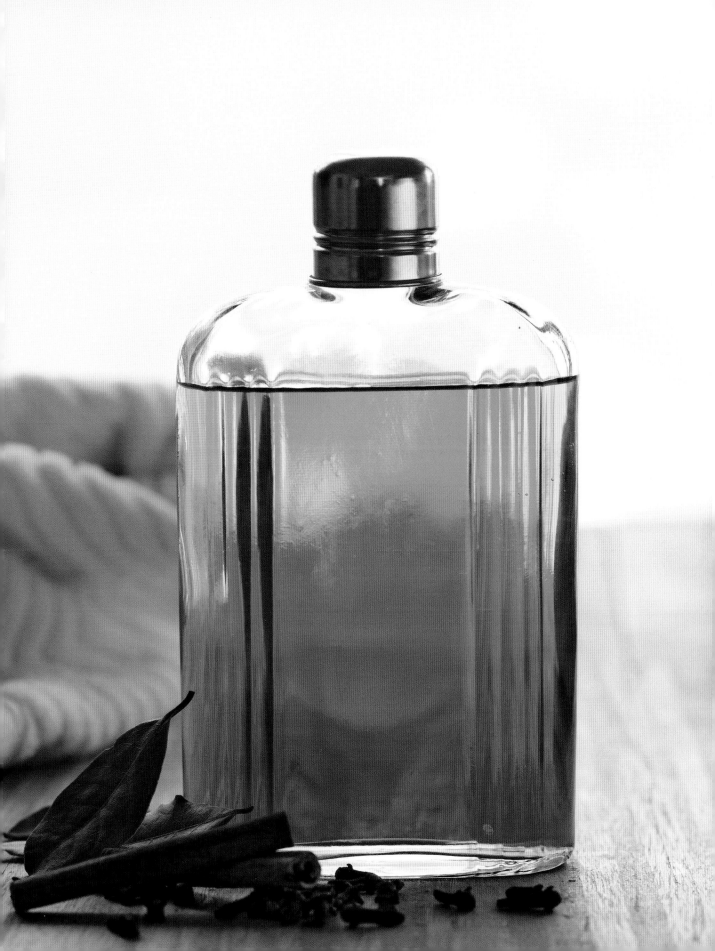

SHAVING BALM

I created this balm with men in mind, but woman can use it as well. It's a healing, moisturizing product that can be used like a shaving cream or applied as a post-shave soother.

YOU WILL NEED:

- ¼ CUP WITCH HAZEL EXTRACT (PURCHASE OR MAKE YOUR OWN BY FOLLOWING THE INSTRUCTIONS FOR MAKING A TINCTURE ON PAGE 74)
- ¼ CUP ALOE VERA GEL
- 1 TABLESPOON GLYCERIN OR HONEY
- BLENDER OR BOWL FOR STIRRING
- 5 TO 10 DROPS TEA TREE ESSENTIAL OIL
- WIDE-MOUTHED CONTAINER WITH LID

(1) Mix the witch hazel, the aloe vera gel, and the glycerin (or honey) thoroughly by hand or with a blender.

(2) Stir in the essential oil, and then transfer the balm to the container.

SPOT TREATMENT FOR PIMPLES

This product works very well as an acute spot treatment. I store it in a mini roller-ball container—the kind that's used for holding perfume. It's great for fighting pimples that are just beginning to form. Simply roll it over the area that needs treating. A little of the spot treatment goes a long way, so I usually make it in very small quantities.

Note: The recipe for this treatment calls for a large quantity of essential oil. Adding jojoba oil infused with sage will make the product even more effective.

YOU WILL NEED:

- ½ TEASPOON LEMON BALM ALCOHOL EXTRACT (FOLLOW THE INSTRUCTIONS FOR MAKING A TINCTURE ON PAGE 74) OR WITCH HAZEL

EXTRACT (PURCHASE OR MAKE YOUR OWN BY FOLLOWING THE INSTRUCTIONS FOR MAKING A TINCTURE ON PAGE 74) OR A COMBINATION OF THE TWO

- ½ TEASPOON JOJOBA OIL
- 10 DROPS LAVENDER ESSENTIAL OIL
- 5 DROPS TEA TREE ESSENTIAL OIL
- 5 DROPS MYRRH ESSENTIAL OIL
- MINI ROLLER-BALL CONTAINER

(1) Pour the lemon balm alcohol extract and the jojoba oil into the roller-ball container.

(2) Add essential oils. Shake before using.

GUEST RECIPE:

JAMIE'S OIL FOR PREMATURE AGING

This salve recipe contributed by my dear friend Jamie, is great for dry and prematurely aging skin. You can substitute half of the apple blossoms with dry rose.

YOU WILL NEED:

- 2 CUPS OF FRESH FORSYTHIA FLOWER, LOOSELY PACKED
- 2 CUPS FRESH APPLE BLOSSOMS
- QUART-SIZED MASON JAR
- 3⅓ TO 3½ CUPS OLIVE OIL

(1) Put the flowers and the blossoms in the jar, and then add the olive oil.

(2) Infuse the mixture over low heat for an hour or two (see Method 2 on page 73), and then strain the flowers.

To use: Take out a month's worth of the oil and keep the rest in the fridge. Don't apply the oil when it's cold. It should be at room temperature when you use it.

LIP BALMS AND CHAPSTICKS

Another product that's easy to whip up in large quantities, a lip treatment makes a great—and much-appreciated—gift. A dear friend of mine can't use commercial balms because they irritate his lips. This is probably due to the chemicals and dyes that are in them. My homemade treatments don't cause him any problems!

Chapstick tubes are an inexpensive and professional-looking way of packaging your lip treatments. For balms that are applied with the finger, use small, wide-mouthed containers. If I make a balm, I alter the chapstick recipe below by using less beeswax (only a table-spoon), which results in a product that spreads more easily. As always, feel free to alter oil ratios and the amount of beeswax to suit your tastes. The recipe below will fill about eight chapstick tubes with a little extra left over.

Citrusy essential oils are good choices for lip treatments, as are peppermint and lavender. Keep in mind that when you're making lip treatments, the less essential oil used the better. Too much essential oil can irritate lips that are sensitive or already chapped.

BASIC CHAPSTICK

YOU WILL NEED:

- GLASS OR PYREX MEASURING CUP
- POT OR SAUCEPAN
- 1 TABLESPOON COCONUT, COCOA BUTTER, OR SHEA BUTTER OIL, SOLID AT ROOM TEMPERATURE
- 2 TABLESPOONS LIQUID OIL (GRAPESEED, JOJOBA, OLIVE, SUNFLOWER, AND AVOCADO ARE GOOD CHOICES)*
- 1 TABLESPOON + 1 TEASPOON GRATED BEESWAX OR BEESWAX PELLETS
- 5 DROPS VITAMIN E OIL (OPTIONAL)
- 5 TO 10 DROPS ESSENTIAL OIL (OPTIONAL)
- 8 CHAPSTICK TUBES

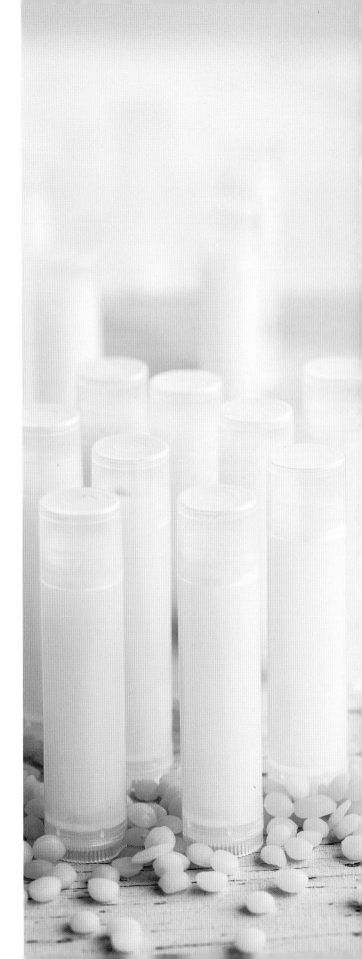

*To make an extra-healing balm for chapped lips, use a calendula- or chickweed-infused liquid oil.

① Create a simple double boiler for warming the ingredients. Put about 2 inches of water into the pot. Then put all of the ingredients except the vitamin E oil and the essential oils in the measuring cup, place the cup in the pot, and heat the water. Make sure it doesn't boil!

② Gently melt the solid oils and the beeswax. Once the beeswax has thoroughly melted, remove it from the heat, and add the vitamin E and the essential oils.

③ Immediately transfer the balm to the containers. If it begins to solidify before you've transferred all of it, put it back in the pot of water and warm it again.

Note: Allow the balm to cool completely in the containers before you cap them. Leave them overnight if necessary to ensure they cool and harden sufficiently.

LAVENDER-HONEY LIP BALM

This soothing, yummy lip balm doubles as a healing treatment for cuts. It can prevent scarring.

● 1 TABLESPOON LAVENDER-INFUSED BASE OIL (TRY GRAPESEED, JOJOBA, OLIVE, SUNFLOWER, OR AVOCADO)

● 1½ TEASPOONS BEESWAX

● 1 TABLESPOON HONEY

● 5 DROPS VITAMIN E OIL (OPTIONAL)

● SMALL CONTAINER WITH LID

① To melt the beeswax in the lavender-infused oil, follow the directions for making a double boiler in the Basic Chapstick recipe on page 113.

② Pour the beeswax lavender mixture into a bowl, and set that bowl in another bowl filled with ice water (like the opposite of a double boiler), to make an ice bath to cool it quicker. Stir in the honey thoroughly and rapidly. Stir in the vitamin E oil if desired.

③ Spoon the balm into the container, and let it sit for at least 2 to 3 hours.

To use: Apply a dab of the balm to your lips with a finger.

FILLING THOSE PESKY LITTLE TUBES!

Filling chapstick tubes can be a tiresome and messy task! To make the process easier, you can purchase trays to hold the tubes. When I use the trays, though, it often seems as if half of my balm ends up on the counter! I usually go with a method suggested to me by a friend: I use an inexpensive, heat-resistant squeeze bottle with a plastic applicator tip (you can find such a bottle at most craft or kitchen stores). I pour the hot chapstick mixture into the bottle and then dispense it into the tubes. This easy method is great for dispensing salves or perfumes into small containers, too.

BODY CARE

LOTIONS, CREAMS, AND BODY BUTTERS

My favorite products to make, hands down, are lotions, body butters, and creams. They're a bit more complicated to put together than some of the other preparations in this book, but the work is worth the effort. The steps involved can seem miraculous at times (in some cases, you're causing oil and water to mix!), and the results are never less than impressive.

With their irresistible scents and inviting textures, these lotions and creams can easily be mistaken for store-bought items. Your friends will be amazed that you made them yourself! And there's a bonus: I find these homemade products to be superior in quality and more moisturizing than anything I've purchased at a store.

In recent years, people have become more knowledgeable about the chemicals and additives used in body-care products, many of which can have unintended effects on the hair and the skin. As a result, the natural body-product business is one of the fastest-growing industries in the country. Unfortunately, though, many of the natural body-care products sold in stores come with their own share of problems:

→ Commercially made natural body-care products are usually more expensive than their additive-filled counterparts. I've often purchased the natural version of a lotion or a shampoo only to find that I spent twice as much on it as I would've on the additive-filled kind.

→ Store-bought products that say they're natural sometimes aren't. Many commercially produced natural products are indeed made with some natural ingredients, but they also contain potentially harmful chemical additives. When I started reading product labels on so-called "natural" products, the number of "unnatural" ingredients listed really surprised me.

WHY SHOULD YOU MAKE YOUR OWN HERBAL BODY-CARE PRODUCTS?

→ **They're surprisingly simple to put together! Some of the easier ones can be made with very little preparation in just a few minutes. The more difficult ones can generally be made in an afternoon or a day.**

→ **They're significantly cheaper than those you purchase in the store. If any of the ingredients called for in this book are out of your price range, you can often find cheaper counterparts.**

→ **They can be made to suit your body's specific needs. These are not one-size-fits-all products! The basic recipes can be amended to fit your body's specific needs. I provide a spectrum of ingredients to suit different skin and hair types.**

→ **You get to choose what goes into the products, so there are no unknown factors involved.**

→ **Many of the oils, vinegars, and herbs the recipes require are probably already in your kitchen. They're quite common and often used in food recipes. That's right—these ingredients are safe enough to eat.**

→ **Making your own body-care products can be fun. And addictive. Trust me— once you start making them, you'll be hooked. You won't want to go back to using the store-bought versions.**

→ Store-bought lotions and creams often come in general, one-size-fits-all formulas, when we know darn well that all bodies are unique and have different needs.

ROSEMARY GLADSTAR'S PERFECT CREAM

Rosemary describes why this recipe has such a special place in her repertoire: My favorite cream by far, this is a product I've made many, many times, always with amazing success.

What makes this cream "perfect"? For starters, it contains a large percentage of water, which is important because dehydration dries out the skin. Any good moisturizing cream should contain plenty of water. The oil in the cream coats, soothes, and protects the skin. Most importantly, though, it holds in the water.

A perfect cream, then, contains an approximately equal balance of water and oil. But because the two don't mix well, getting them to cohabitate in a cream is tricky. For this reason, the recipe can be a bit challenging. Just follow the instructions closely, and if the cream doesn't turn out right the first time, don't be discouraged. Try it again! This luscious product is worth the work.

YOU WILL NEED:

- 2/3 CUP DISTILLED WATER* (OR ROSE WATER)
- 1/3 CUP ALOE VERA GEL
- 1 OR 2 DROPS ESSENTIAL OIL OF CHOICE
- VITAMINS A AND E AS DESIRED

- 3/4 CUPS APRICOT, ALMOND, OR GRAPESEED OIL
- 1/3 CUP COCONUT OIL OR COCOA BUTTER
- 1/4 TEASPOON LANOLIN
- 1/2 TO 1 OUNCE GRATED BEESWAX

- GLASS MEASURING CUP
- DOUBLE BOILER OR POT
- BLENDER
- SEVERAL CREAM OR LOTION JARS WITH LIDS

*Tap water can be used instead of distilled water, but it will sometimes introduce bacteria and encourage the growth of mold.

1. Pour the first four ingredients, from water through vitamins A and E, into a glass measuring cup. Set aside.

2. Combine the remaining four ingredients in a double boiler (you can make your own double boiler by following the instructions in the Basic Chapstick recipe on page 113), and warm over low heat until melted.

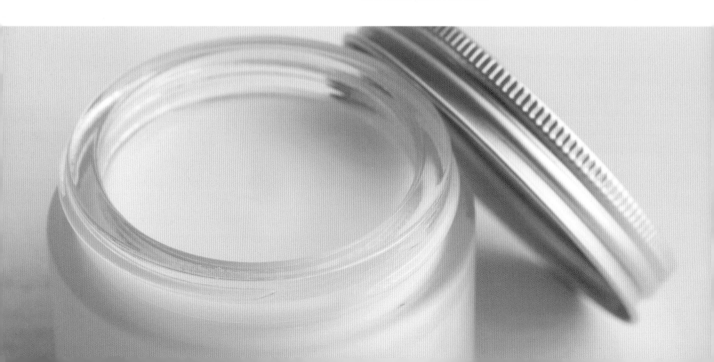

③ Pour the oils into the blender and let them cool to room temperature. The mixture should become thick, creamy, semisolid, and cream colored. To speed up the cooling process, put the oils in the refrigerator, but keep an eye on them and make sure they don't become too hard.

④ When the mixture has cooled, turn on the blender at its highest speed. Pour the water mixture slowly (in a thin trickle) into the center vortex of the whirling oil mixture.

⑤ Once most of the water mixture has been added to the oils, listen to the blender and watch the cream. When the machine coughs and chokes and the cream looks thick and white (like buttercream frosting), turn the blender off. You can slowly add more water, beating it in by hand with a spoon, but don't overbeat! The cream will thicken as it sets.

⑥ Pour the mixture into glass cream or lotion jars, and store them in a cool location. They don't need to be refrigerated.

Rosemary Gladstar's Perfect Cream should never become moldy or go bad. If it does, it's probably due to one or more of the following reasons:

→ Recycled Lids. If you reuse a container, be sure the inner cardboard ring in the lid has been removed. It's a perfect host for bacteria.

→ Food Ingredients. Many foods support bacterial growth. For instance, if you blend frozen strawberries into your cream base because you want the product to have a strawberry scent, your cream will develop mold within days.

→ Improper storage. Make sure the cream stays cool. Don't store it in a warm location. Keep any extra cream you have in the refrigerator or in a cool pantry. If you live in a hot climate, refrigeration can extend the cream's shelf life.

Tips for Making and Using Rosemary Gladstar's Perfect Cream

For many years, when I made this cream, I put the waters into the blender first and then added the oils. One day, one of my students told me she reversed the process and never encountered any problems with separation between the waters and the oil. Simple suggestions like hers have made the cream successful and enduring. So I encourage you to experiment and play with the recipe.

Unlike many commercial products that only coat the surface of the skin, this cream penetrates the surface and moisturizes the skin's dermal layer. Because it's extremely concentrated, a little goes a long way. A tiny drop on the end of your finger is all you need. Gently massage the cream into your face. There will be a temporary feeling of oiliness, but it will disappear within a few minutes as the cream is absorbed. I recommend using a small amount on your face, but you can apply the cream generously to the rest of your body.

There's only one real "rule" regarding this cream: When using it, you must think only positive thoughts about your body and yourself. Banish the negative! Apply the cream to your skin with love, as though you're anointing yourself with a precious balm, because you are! That's part of the cream's magic.

If you follow the recipe precisely, the cream should turn out well. If the waters and oils separate, they probably weren't at the right temperature. The waters should be at room temperature, and the oils should be completely cool. If the waters and oils separate, then start over. Or just put a little note that says "Shake Before Using" on the finished bottle of cream.

EMOLLIENT BODY BUTTER

Thick, rich, and moisturizing, this body butter is great for extremely dry skin and can help with conditions such as eczema and psoriasis.

YOU WILL NEED:

- ½ CUP COCOA BUTTER
- ½ CUP COCONUT OIL
- POT OR SAUCEPAN
- 4 TABLESPOONS ALOE VERA GEL
- 1 TABLESPOON SHEA BUTTER
- 1 TABLESPOON AVOCADO OIL
- 1 TABLESPOON JOJOBA OIL
- ¼ TEASPOON VITAMIN E LIQUID IN CAPSULE FORM
- 25 DROPS ESSENTIAL OIL (TRY LAVENDER OR A CITRUS OIL)
- WIDE-MOUTHED JAR WITH LID

1. Melt the cocoa butter and coconut oil over very low heat in a clean pot, stirring occasionally until they've completely melted.

2. Stir in the remaining ingredients except for the essential oil.

3. Remove the pot from the heat, add the essential oil, and mix the ingredients thoroughly by hand or with a mixer or blender.

4. Transfer the body butter to the jar. It will thicken and solidify in the coming days.

To use: The body butter works best when used right after a bath or shower on moist skin. It'll seal in the moisture.

SUPER BODY BUTTER

This easy recipe makes an emollient body butter that's extremely healing for dry, cracked skin. It's wonderful for the elbows and feet. It can also be used as a shaving butter.

YOU WILL NEED:

- 1 CUP COCONUT OIL
- ½ CUP SHEA BUTTER
- 2 TABLESPOONS HONEY
- 1 TABLESPOON ALOE VERA GEL
- 25 DROPS BERGAMOT OIL (OR OTHER CITRUS OIL)
- WIDE-MOUTHED JAR WITH LID

1. Blend all of the ingredients thoroughly either by hand in a pot or with a blender or mixer.

2. Once the mixture is smooth, transfer it to the jar. It will thicken and solidify in the coming days.

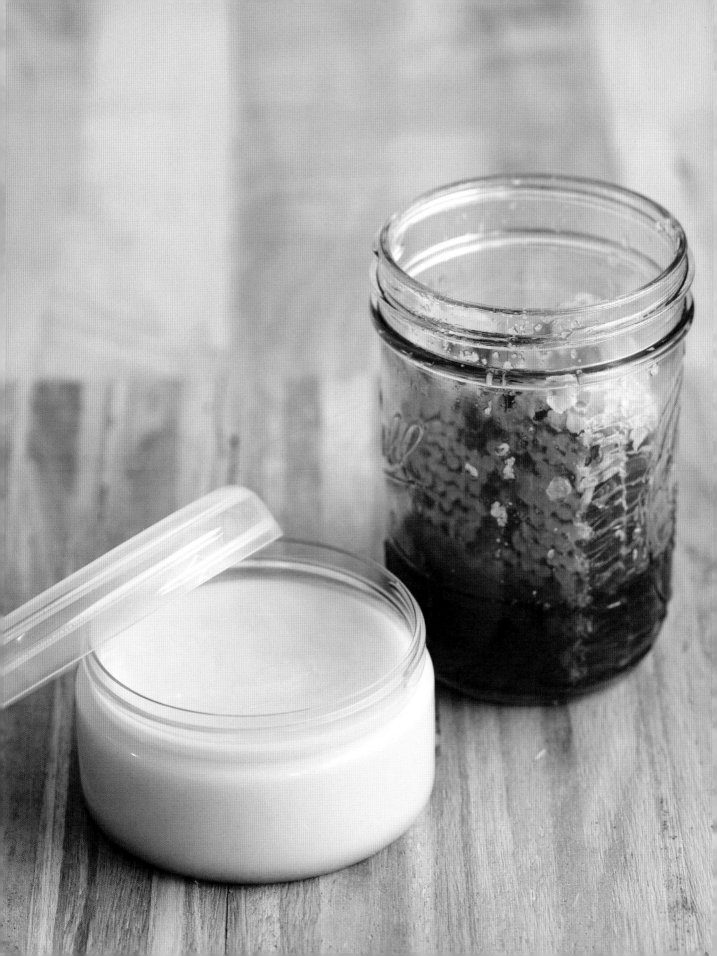

OIL FOR WEATHERED, SCARRED, OR AGED SKIN

This nutrient-rich liquid oil provides nourishment for aged and weathered skin. It can help reduce fine lines and wrinkles, and diminish the appearance of scars. *Note:* You may find the scent a bit overpowering because of the flax oil.

YOU WILL NEED:

- 2 TABLESPOONS ARGON OIL
- 2 TABLESPOONS FLAX OIL
- 2 TABLESPOONS WHEAT GERM OIL
- 2 TABLESPOONS BORAGE OIL
- 20 DROPS FRANKINCENSE AND/OR YLANG YLANG ESSENTIAL OIL
- BOWL
- SQUEEZE BOTTLE

Mix the oils together in a bowl, and then transfer them to the squeeze bottle.

To use: Warm a bit of the oil in your hands and apply it at bedtime. It will nourish your skin overnight. Keep the oil refrigerated so that it doesn't spoil.

DEODORANT

We've all heard that commercial deodorants may contain harmful chemicals. Making your own is an easy and effective alternative. This recipe makes a liquid deodorant. The antibacterial properties of the herbs help to control unwanted odors, and the essential oils add a lovely scent.

For storage, try reusing an old liquid deodorant container. You can also put the deodorant in a spray bottle or apply it with a cotton ball.

YOU WILL NEED:

- ½ CUP SAGE ALCOHOL EXTRACT (FOLLOW THE INSTRUCTIONS FOR MAKING A TINCTURE ON PAGE 74) OR WITCH HAZEL EXTRACT (PURCHASE OR MAKE YOUR OWN BY FOLLOWING THE INSTRUCTIONS FOR MAKING A TINCTURE ON PAGE 74)
- 1 TEASPOON GLYCERIN
- 30 DROPS MYRRH ESSENTIAL OIL
- 25 DROPS ESSENTIAL OIL(S) OF YOUR CHOICE (TRY PEPPERMINT, LAVENDER, YLANG YLANG, OR ROSEMARY)
- BOWL
- STORAGE CONTAINER OF YOUR CHOICE

Mix the ingredients together thoroughly in the bowl, and then transfer the deodorant to the container.

To use: Shake the deodorant before you use it. Apply daily as needed.

PERFUMES

I love perfumes! The scents we choose to wear say a lot about who we are. They reflect our personalities. Perfumes are also powerful mood boosters. They have the ability to lift the spirit.

Playing with and mixing fragrances can be something of an adventure. When you make your own perfumes, you have the ability to create something entirely new. Making them is easy and fun. It's also a great way to experiment with and learn about your essential oils. I like to get creative with my essential-oil perfumes and add small crystals or glitter to them. The sparkly bottles of sweet-smelling stuff make great gifts.

I use a lot of essential oils in my perfumes. If they're too strong for you, feel free to experiment and use smaller amounts. For storage, use small roller-ball bottles.

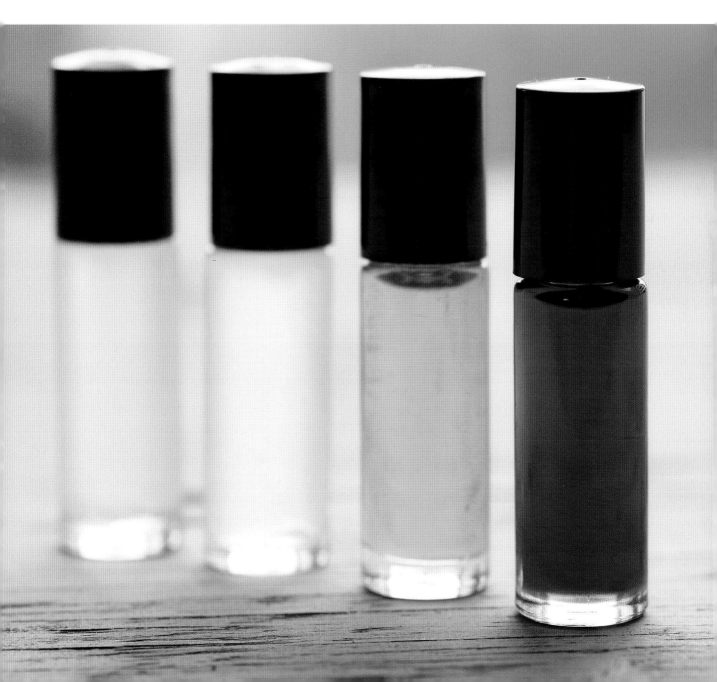

LIQUID ROLL-ON PERFUME

YOU WILL NEED:

- 1 TEASPOON CARRIER OIL (I USE GRAPESEED, AS IT HAS NO SCENT. CANOLA AND SOY CAN ALSO BE USED.)
- 40 DROPS ESSENTIAL OIL OR COMBINATION OF ESSENTIAL OILS
- 1 TO 2 DROPS ALCOHOL (TRY RUBBING ALCOHOL, VODKA, OR GIN. I USE AN EYEDROPPER FOR THIS STEP. DON'T FILL THE DROPPER; JUST PICK UP A COUPLE OF DROPS.)
- SMALL ROLLER-BALL CONTAINER
- GLITTER OR CRYSTALS (OPTIONAL)

(1) Pour the carrier oil into the roller-ball container. Add the essential oil(s), the alcohol, and the glitter or crystals, if desired.

(2) Put the roller-ball top on the container, and shake the perfume well.

HENNA FOR BODY DECORATION

Body painting with natural pigments and plant dyes was once a common practice in cultures around the world. It was a ritual done in preparation for births, weddings, funerals, and war. Henna has a long history of this type of ritualistic use. It was popular among the ancient Egyptians, who also used it for cosmetic purposes.

Today, painting the body is a way to connect with the customs of the past. I recently had my hands hennaed as part of a wedding ceremony. The groom was from India, and the use of henna at weddings is a tradition in his country. It was a beautiful, powerful ritual that I felt lucky to be a part of.

Henna decoration can be a fun party activity. (It's neat to think about the past generations of people who have done the very same thing!)

The easiest way to use it is to purchase a henna kit. Patterns can be painted on freehand or with the aid of stencils. If you purchase henna powder, you can mix your own henna paste, but this can be time-consuming. Make sure you consult the directions that accompany your kit. To apply the henna, you can use a plastic baggie with a tip applicator or a baggie with the tip cut off. You can also purchase henna applicators, and many kits come with them.

HENNA RECIPE

YOU WILL NEED:

- ¼ CUP DRIED HENNA LEAF POWDER
- 1 CUP LEMON JUICE (FRESH OR BOTTLED)
- 1½ TEASPOONS SUGAR (PREMIXED HENNA POWDERS DON'T REQUIRE THIS; CHECK THE DIRECTIONS)
- APPLICATOR

(1) Mix the henna powder and the lemon juice until the mixture is smooth. Then stir in the sugar (if required), and mix until smooth.

(2) Let the henna sit for a while to make sure the dye is released. The longer you let it sit, the stronger its color will be when you apply it. You can let it sit for a few hours or overnight.

(3) Mix the henna again until it's smooth. If it's thick, add a little more lemon juice.

(4) Transfer the henna to the applicator.

Tip: Once you apply the henna, it will begin to dry. The longer you keep it moist, the more intense the color will become. Use tea tree oil and lemon juice to keep it moist. The henna will get darker the longer you leave it on. (I've left henna on overnight before.) It will flake off as it dries. Once it's dry, you can easily brush or wash it off. You'll be left with a lovely auburn-orange body decoration.

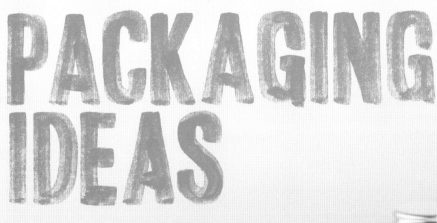

PACKAGING IDEAS

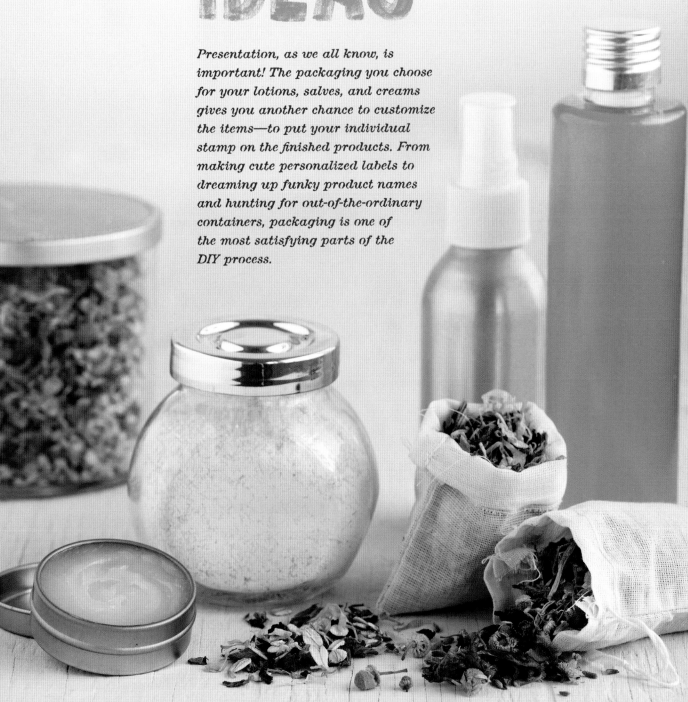

Presentation, as we all know, is important! The packaging you choose for your lotions, salves, and creams gives you another chance to customize the items—to put your individual stamp on the finished products. From making cute personalized labels to dreaming up funky product names and hunting for out-of-the-ordinary containers, packaging is one of the most satisfying parts of the DIY process.

MAKING LABELS

Labeling your products, even if they're only for personal use, is important for a number of reasons. You may think you'll remember what a product is and what its ingredients are, but I can confirm from personal experience that once some time has passed, it's often difficult to remember the details regarding a specific item, especially when you have three (or more) unlabeled jars in your bathroom.

Labeling is even more important if your products are serving as gifts. When I give my products to others, I make labels for each of them with information about ingredients and usage. I use inexpensive sticker labels that can be found at most craft or office-supply stores. These labels can be written on by hand or printed on using a computer—a smart option if you're going for a professional look or need multiple labels for an individual product. I usually handwrite my labels, but printing them is much easier.

Fancy handmade paper, colored paper, and notecards also make lovely labels for products that you can't stick a sticker on. Wallpaper samples are another pretty, inexpensive substitute. I often cut fun shapes out of paper, punch holes in them, and thread string through so that I can tie the labels to the products.

Naming Your Products

I find that inventing creative, humorous names for my products can be lots of fun! Names also add a touch of professionalism and legitimacy to the entire enterprise. When I'm making something for a specific person, I usually try to come up with a name that I know he or she will get a kick out of or find significant.

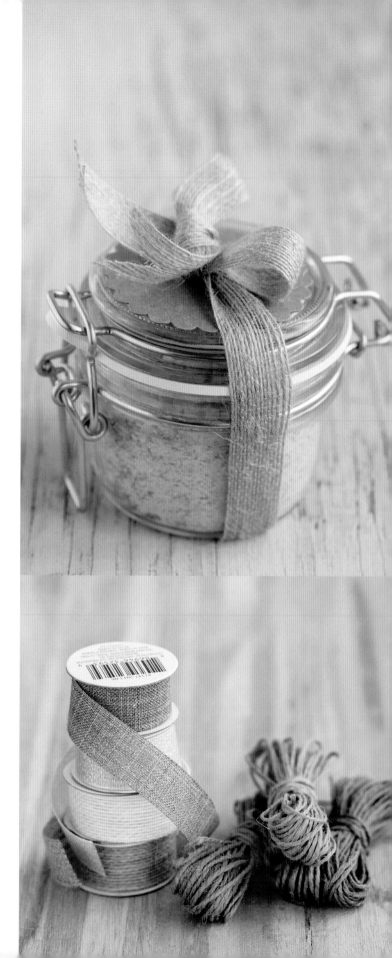

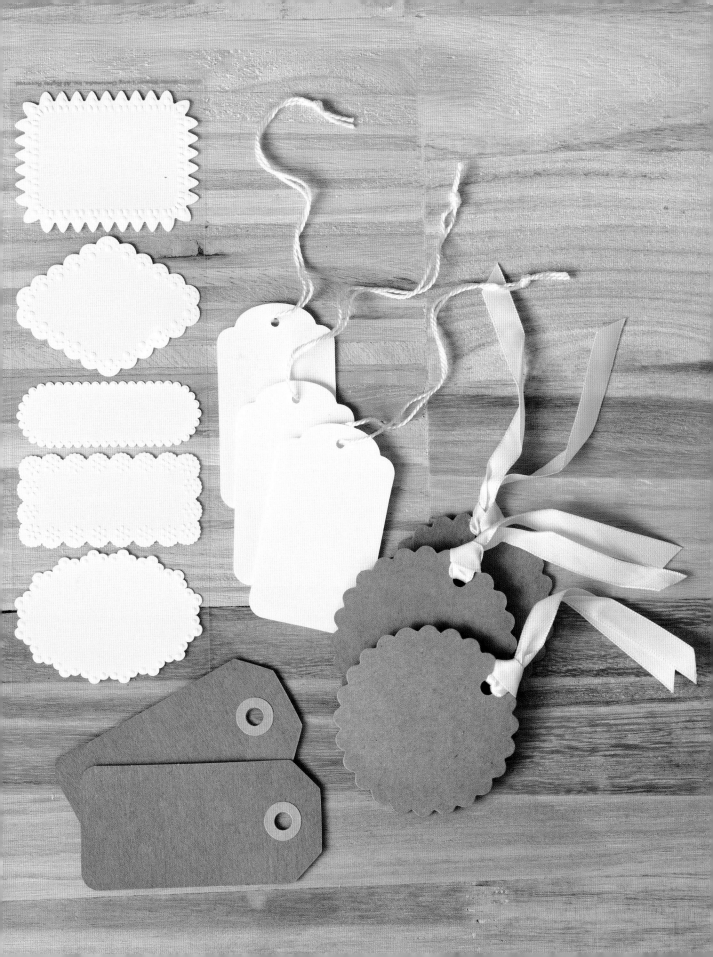

CONTAINERS

Whether your taste runs to traditional glass jars or out-of-the-ordinary vessels, you can make a statement with the containers you choose for your products. Craft stores offer lots of neat options, and bottles in all shapes and sizes, including cute glass receptacles for salves, pump containers for lotions, and squeeze bottles for shampoos, can be ordered online from bath- and beauty-supply websites.

I also visit thrift shops when I'm in need of interesting containers for my products. The search can be very rewarding, and the items are cheap. I like to use glass containers in colors like cobalt blue, green, and brown. These vessels make lovely gifts and are great for holding products made with oils that are sensitive to light.

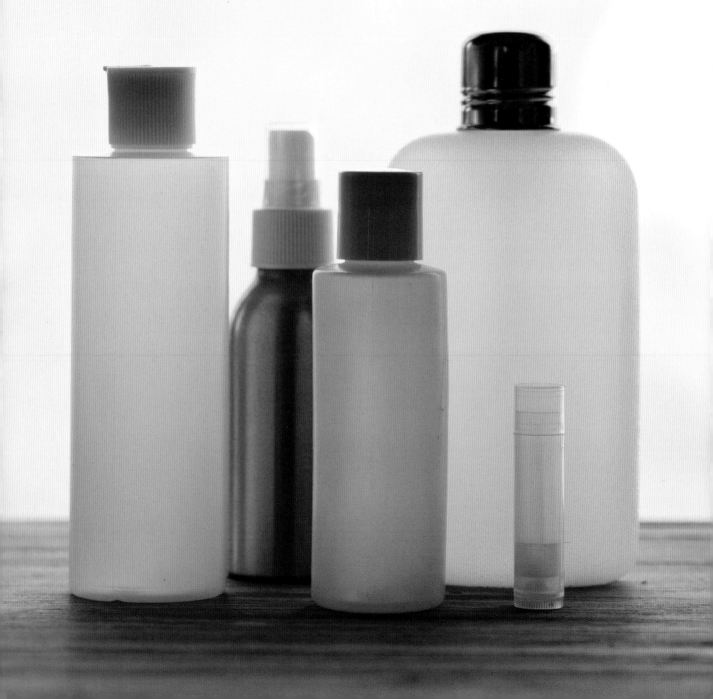

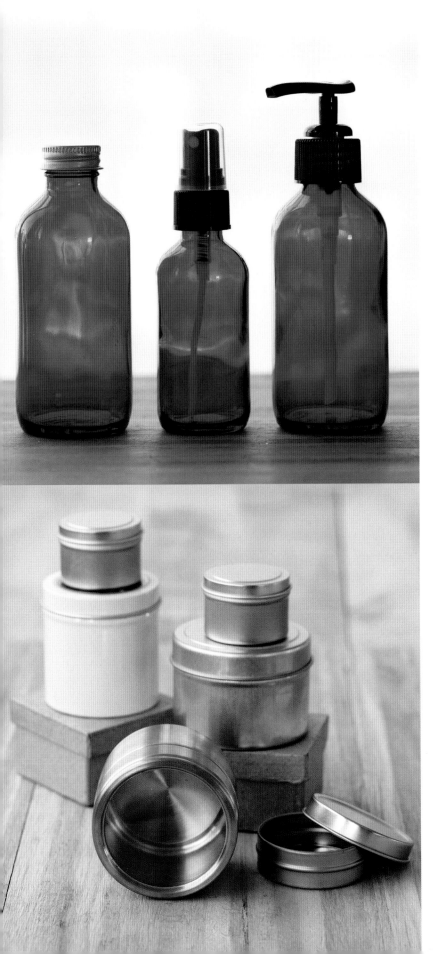

The old-fashioned canning jar—the kind with the metal lid that your grandma probably used—is a favorite among herbalists. This type of jar is perfect for making herbal alcohol, glycerin, and oil extracts, and it's a great storage container for dried herbs. Canning jars also make cute vessels for products such as lotions and bath salts. Try covering the tops of the metal lids with squares of fabric like grandma used to when she gave canned goodies to friends.

Small plastic bags are useful for holding dry facial masks and scrubs, bath salts, and herbal bath soaks. They're convenient and cheap.

Small cloth pouches for holding bath salts and soaks that contain plant matter can be found at most craft stores or purchased from one of the venders listed in the Additional Resources section on page 139. Cloth pouches are available in bulk. They're usually made of muslin and have a simple drawstring. If you have minimal sewing skills (or a sewing machine), you can easily make them at home. Other options include clean socks and feet cut from pantyhose or tights (colored tights are fun to use), which can be repurposed as pouches. You can reuse all of the pouches—simply turn them inside out, dispose of the plant matter (compost, please!), rinse out the pouch, and let it dry.

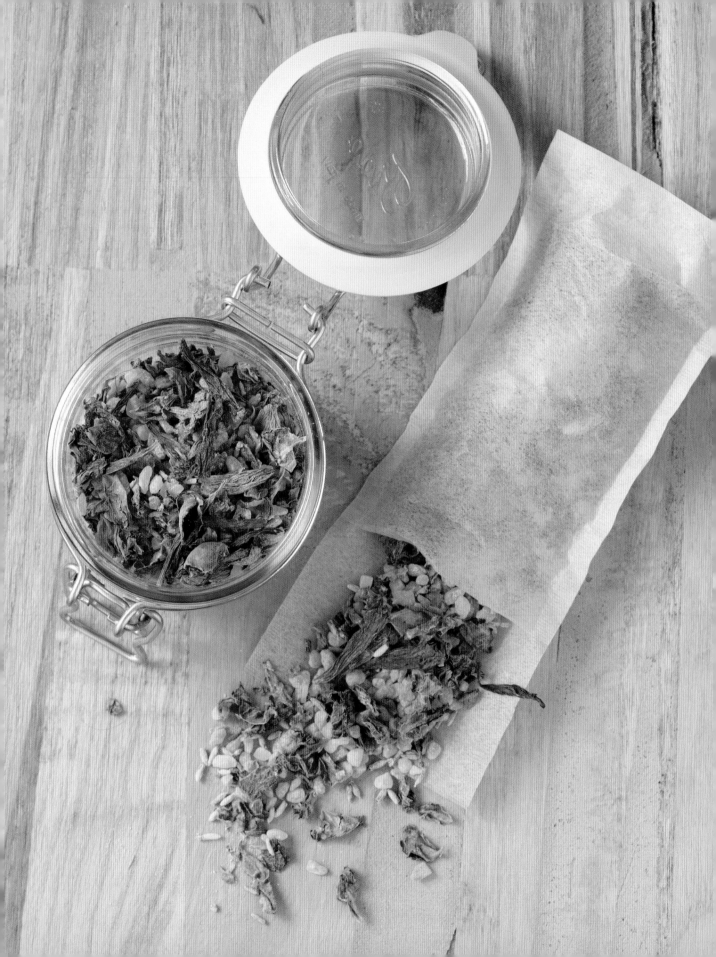

Tea filters function like tea bags in the bath. The filters can be filled with bath salts and soaks, so when they're placed in the bath the scent and benefits of their herbal contents are released, but they don't leave any plant residue. It's a good thing to keep in mind when you're giving bath salts and soaks as gifts.

Reusing Containers

Some makers of herbal products feel it's a bad idea to reuse containers, especially if they will hold creams or lotions made with oils that could go rancid or cause mold to grow. It's true that reused containers can harbor bacteria and fungus if they're not cleaned well. Also, many containers have lids with cardboard rings inside. If you're reusing a container with such a lid, remove the cardboard! It's impossible to clean, and it can harbor bacteria.

That said, I've reused many a container and never had a problem. When I reuse a bottle or jar, I wash it thoroughly in very hot water. If I have extra doubts about a container (if it's a thrift-store purchase, for instance), I wipe it out with alcohol to kill any germs. As a general rule, unless a container is sealed when purchased, I wash it.

Repurposing containers you already have is another way to save money. I've repurposed jars that have held everything from peanut butter to olives. Glass baby-food jars are great for repurposing. Olive-oil dispensers or bottles that have held oils also make attractive containers. If you have an interesting glass jar you'd like to repurpose, clean it thoroughly. If it has a label that needs to be removed, soak it in soapy hot water overnight. The label should come right off. A jar with a stubborn label should be soaked in kitchen oil.

A few tips: Chapstick tubes, perfume bottles, and shampoo bottles can all be reused. Just make sure you clean them as thoroughly as possible. If you're packaging a product that will be used in the shower, go with a plastic container—you'll be eliminating the risk of an accident involving broken glass. Many containers, including chapstick tubes and roller-ball bottles, are available in bulk. Suppliers of bulk containers are listed in the Resources section on page 139. If you're in need of unique containers and jars for packaging, ask your friends to be on the lookout and save them for you.

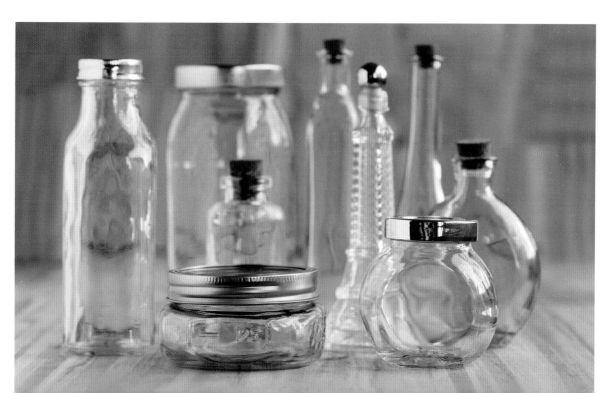

GIFT BASKETS

Gift baskets filled with personalized body-care products make great gifts for friends and family. They're perfect for holiday giving, special occasions, and birthdays. Once again, the possibilities for packaging are endless: Try putting the products in an actual basket, covering it with colored plastic wrap or tissue paper, and adding a ribbon. You can also use paper or cloth gift bags.

Collect the following items so that you have plenty of options when it comes time to package your products:

- STICKER LABELS
- HANDMADE PAPER
- WALLPAPER SAMPLES
- COLORED PAPER
- INTERESTING PAPER SCRAPS
- BITS OF STRING OR COLORED RIBBON
- FABRIC SCRAPS
- CANNING JARS IN VARIOUS SIZES
- REPURPOSED CONTAINERS AND JARS THAT YOU FIND INTERESTING
- PLASTIC BAGGIES
- DECORATIVE BOTTLES WITH CORKS
- OLIVE-OIL DISPENSERS
- SMALL CLOTH POUCHES
- COMPUTER AND PRINTER OR FUN PENS FOR WRITING LABELS

Here are a few of my favorite gift-basket ideas. Give one of them a try or make up your own using products you've designed for a friend's specific needs. Be creative!

Ultimate Face Care
Great for people with problem skin

Basic Clay Mask (personalized) and/or Herbal-Honey Facial Mask

Rosemary Gladstar's Perfect Cream

Rosemary Gladstar's Miracle Grains

Astringent or Toner (personalized)

Spot Treatment for Pimples (optional)

Lavender-Honey Lip Balm or Basic Chapstick

The Athlete's Friend
Relief for sore muscles and other issues

Icy-Hot Foot Salve

Arnica Salve for Pain and Bruises

Epsom Salt Sore-Muscle Soak

Wake-Up Bath Soak

Deodorant

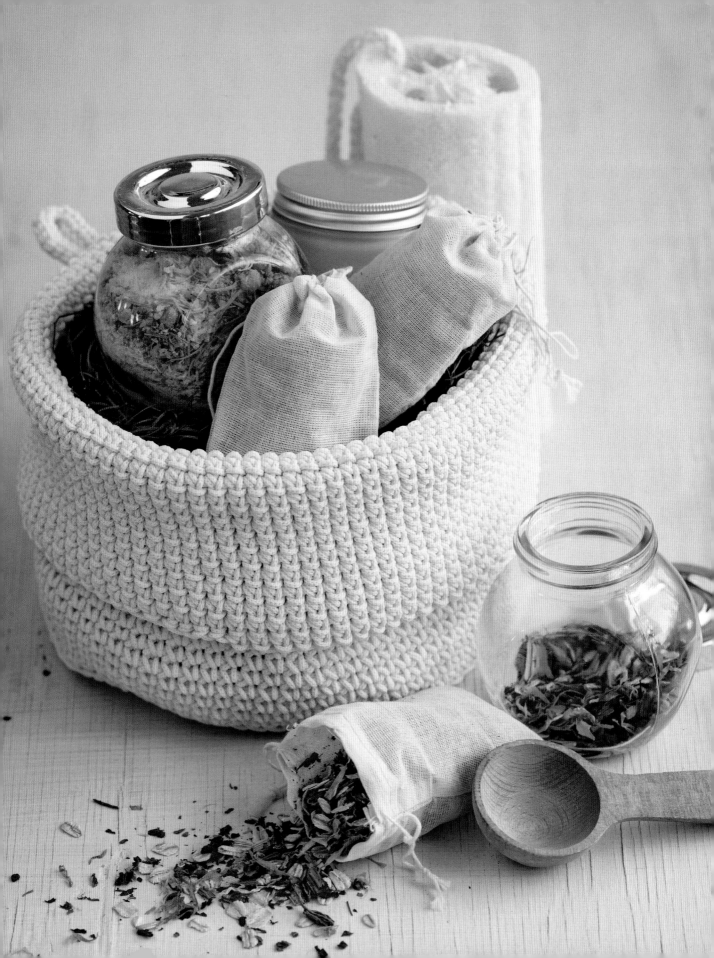

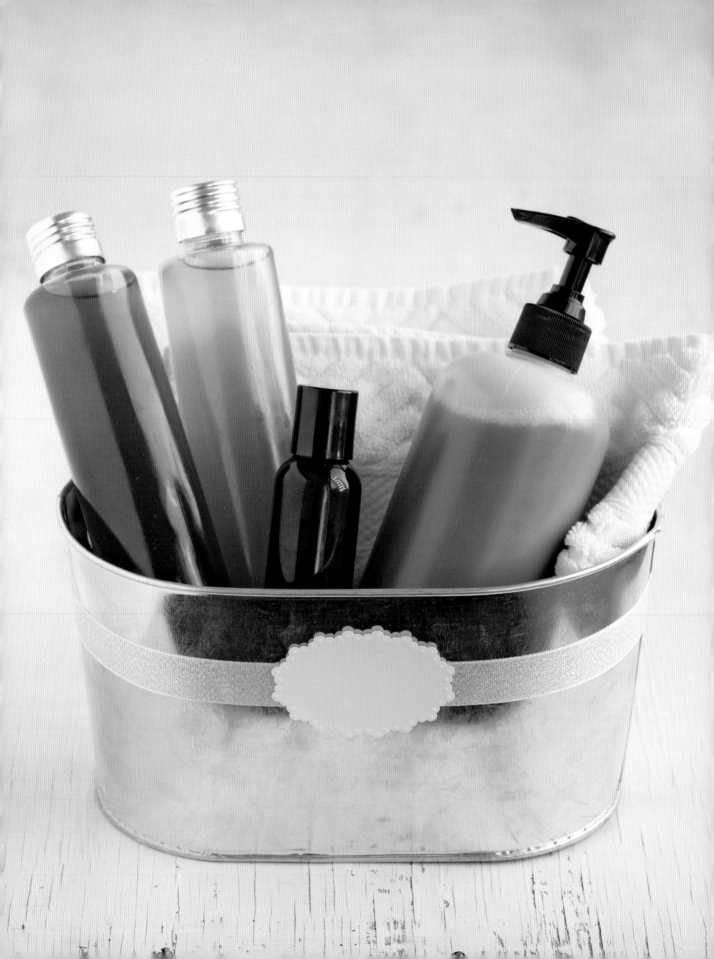

Luxurious Locks

Everything you need for
a beautiful head of hair

**Shampoo
(personalized)**

**Dried herbs for herbal hair
rinse with directions for use**

**Conditioning oil treatment
(personalized)**

Salt Hair Volumizer

**Lemon-Coconut Hair
Lightener (optional)**

Summer Fun in the Sun

Perfect for a summer vacation

Sunscreen

St. John's Wort Sunburn Salve

Bug Repellent

Salt Hair Volumizer

Lemon-Coconut Hair Lightener

**Bath Soak for Rashes,
Bug Bites, or Dry Skin**

Manly Face Care

A basket of goodies that
have a masculine scent

Bay Rum Aftershave and Toner

Shaving Balm

**Spot Treatment for Pimples
(optional)**

Basic Chapstick

**Rosemary Gladstar's
Perfect Cream**

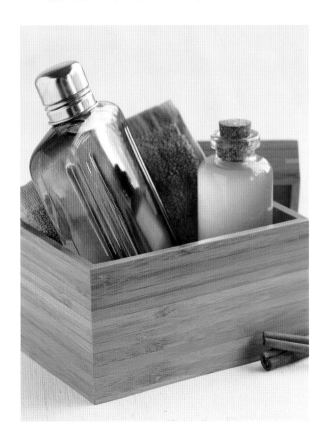

QUICK GIFTS

Most of the body products in this book make amazingly quick, cheap, and beautiful gifts. Many of these projects can be made in less than half an hour and/or in large quantities, which can be divided up for multiple gifts. Products such as those pictured here: bath salts and soaks, face masks, and lip balms make for especially easy, beautiful, and personal gifts. With the addition of some lovely packaging elements such as ribbons, tags, and fancy jars or bags, you have instant memorable presents! There's no doubt your friends and family will be impressed that you made these body products—especially when they use them and see and feel the results.

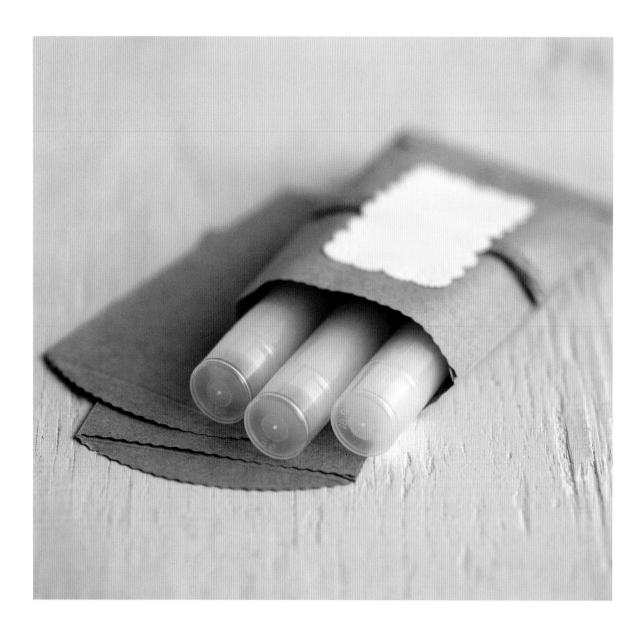

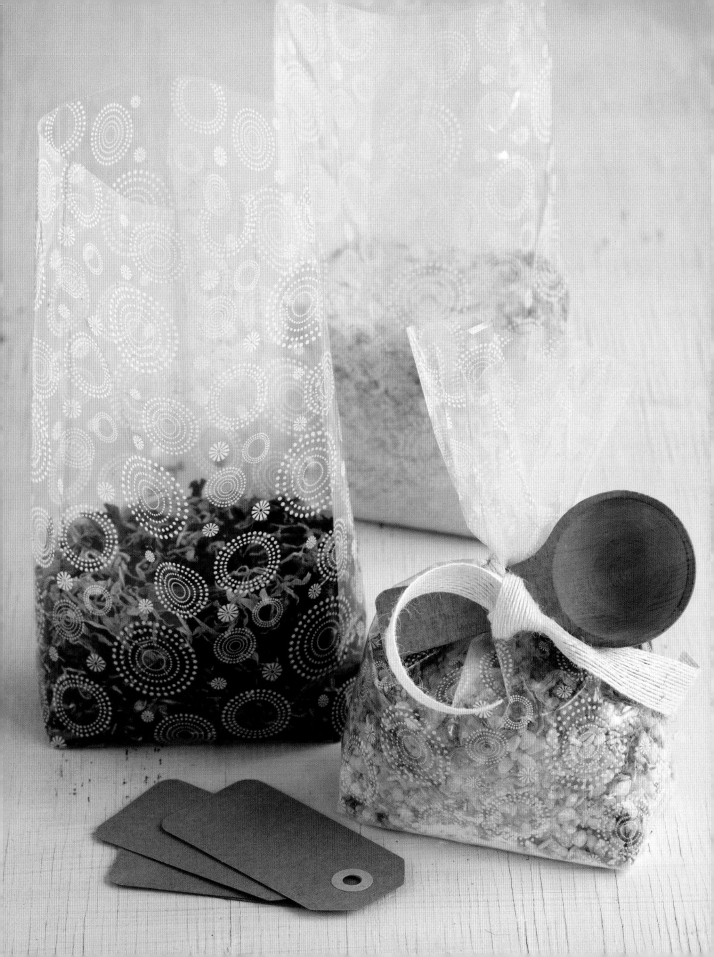

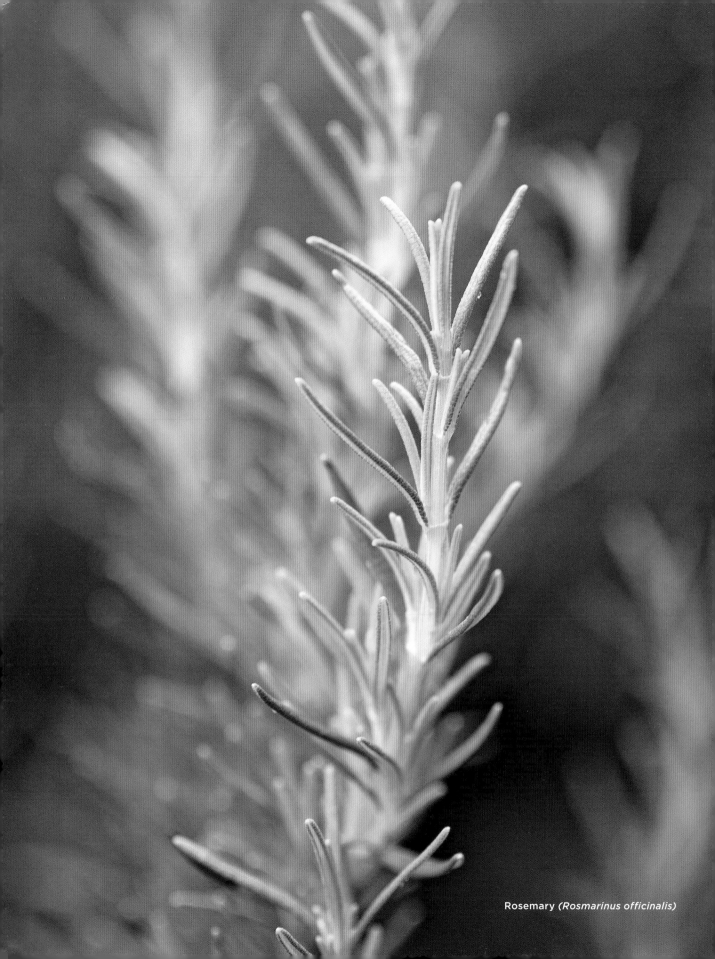

Rosemary *(Rosmarinus officinalis)*

GUEST CONTRIBUTORS

Amy Branum

Amy is a dancer and mother who finds daily inspiration in the beauty of life and the magic of plants. She holds a degree in biology and studied herbalism with Peggy Ellis at what is now the Appalachia School of Holistic Herbalism in Asheville, North Carolina. An herbalist, flower-essence practitioner, and Ayurvedic specialist, Amy shares her love of herbal remedies through her companies Boutique Botanika and Savoir.

Jamie Francisco

A native of New York's Catskill region, which she still calls home, Jamie studied traditional herbalism through the Appalachia School of Holistic Herbalism in Asheville, North Carolina. She furthered her skills at the Blue Ridge School of Herbal Medicine in Weaverville, North Carolina, where she participated in an internship and worked with clients at a free herbal clinic. A farmer, builder, and herbalist who has been foraging and wildcrafting for almost 10 years, Jamie looks forward to one day opening a free clinic in the western Catskills.

Rosemary Gladstar

Rosemary has been teaching and writing about herbs for more than 40 years. She is the author of 10 books, including Rosemary Gladstar's Medicinal Herbs: A Beginner's Guide: 33 Healing Herbs to Know, Grow, and Use; Herbal Healing for Women; and Rosemary Gladstar's Herbal Recipes for Vibrant Health. She is the founder and director of the Sage Mountain Herbal Retreat Center and Botanical Sanctuary, a 500-acre preserve in central Vermont. She is also the founding president of United Plant Savers, the director of the International Herb Symposium, and cofounder of the Traditional Medicinal Tea Company. Rosemary lives and works at the Sage Mountain Herbal Retreat Center.

Toyia Hatten

As a holistic herbalist and herbal educator, Toyia helps others incorporate healing herbs into their everyday lives. She urges others to cultivate a deep connection with the natural world as a way of reducing stress. Toyia grew up in a family of avid plant lovers, and she studied herbalism formally at the Appalachia School of Holistic Herbalism in Asheville, North Carolina. After several plant-filled years in North Carolina, Toyia moved to Montana, where she now shares her love of nature and herbs with a great community of people and explores the beautiful Rocky Mountains.

Amanda Sue Houdek

An experienced chef and chocolatier, Amanda enjoys growing medicinal herbs and incorporating them creatively into her cooking. She holds a baking and pastry degree and has studied with world-renowned chocolate and sugar artists. Amanda studied herbalism informally for seven years and assisted her sister, Heather, in teaching a medicine-making course. Using her knowledge of food alchemy, she loves to create her own herbal body and bath products.

ADDITIONAL RESOURCES

I hope my book inspires you to pursue herbs with passion! To provide you with options for further exploration of the topic, I put together the following list of my favorite resources.

REFERENCE MATERIAL

These amazing titles contain additional information about herbs and the ways they can be used internally for medicinal purposes.

An Ancient Egyptian Herbal
by **Lise Manniche**
(British Museum Press, 2006)
This terrific title puts herbalism's long history into perspective. It covers the plants, recipes, and remedies used by the ancient Egyptians and has an informative section on perfume.

A Field Guide to Medicinal Plants and Herbs: Of Eastern and Central North America (Peterson Field Guides)
by **Steven Foster** and **James A. Duke**
(Houghton Mifflin Harcourt, 1999)
With more than 500 entries, this wonderful guide is indispensible when it comes to identifying and harvesting plants for medicinal purposes.

The Green Pharmacy: The Ultimate Compendium of Natural Remedies from the World's Foremost Authority on Healing Herbs
by **James A. Duke**
(St. Martin's, 1998)
From folk remedies to modern, scientific formulas, this useful book contains more than 100 herbal treatments for health problems.

Healing Wise
by **Susan S. Weed**
(Ash Tree Publishing, 2003)
This little herbal guide brims with helpful information. It provides an in-depth look at a variety of herbs that are probably growing in your yard right now.

The Herbal Medicine-Maker's Handbook: A Home Manual
by **James Green**
(Crossing Press, 2000)
If you want to explore the world of home-made herbal medicines, this is the book for you. It covers everything from gathering and growing herbs to instructions on how to make herbal products.

Rosemary Gladstar's Family Herbal: A Guide to Living Life with Energy, Health, and Vitality
by **Rosemary Gladstar**
(Storey, 2001)
My all-time favorite herbal book, this beautiful title provides an overview of herbs. It also contains a batch of wonderful recipes and a variety of treatment suggestions for both chronic and acute problems.

ORGANIZATIONS

The American Herbalists Guild
americanherbalistsguild.com
The American Herbalists Guild is a great organization to join for those interested in herbal medicine. It was founded in 1989 as a non-profit, educational organization to represent the goals and voices of herbalists specializing in the medicinal use of plants. The website contains lists of member schools and information about mentoring; you may wish to explore it further if you're drawn to follow the path of an herbal education.

United Plant Savers

unitedplantsavers.org

UPS is an incredible nonprofit member organization for anyone interested in herbalism. Their mission statements says, "Our mission is to protect native medicinal plants of the United States and Canada and their native habitat, while ensuring an abundant, renewable supply of medicinal plants for generations to come." The website has a wealth of information regarding conservation of endangered medicinal plants (some of which are featured in this book).

HERBS & HERBAL PRODUCTS

Most of the ingredients in this book can be purchased from your local co-op or natural-food store. If you can't find them there, then try one of the sources below. All are reliable suppliers of herbs, essential oils, and other items.

Floracopeia

floracopeia.com

Floracopeia stocks high-quality essential oils that are sustainably manufactured and harvested. Their website has lots of great information about essential oils and aromatherapy, as well as resources for online study.

Frontier Natural Products Co-op

frontiercoop.com

Frontier is a great source for high-quality herbs, essential oils, additives, recipes, and helpful information.

Mountain Rose Herbs

mountainroseherbs.com

An excellent national supplier of high-quality herbs, essential oils, additives, containers, and ready-made herbal products, Mountain Rose is also a great source of helpful information.

Red Moon Herbs

redmoonherbs.com

Located in western North Carolina, Red Moon Herbs has a small selection of herbs, but they're sustainably harvested and of very good quality.

SEED SUPPLIERS

Baker Creek Heirloom Seeds

rareseeds.com

Located in Missouri, this is a wonderful, ethical source for heirloom seeds. All the seeds are non-hybrid, non-GMO, non-treated, and non-patented.

Horizon Herbs

horizonherbs.com

Located in Oregon, this small company is a diverse, wholesome source for medicinal herb seeds and plants. They have a wonderful selection!

Seed Savers Exchange

seedsavers.org

Located in Iowa, this is a nonprofit dedicated to preserving heirloom seeds and biodiversity. It is funded through donations and seed sales. They have interesting heirloom seeds including a great herb selection—one of my favorite places to purchase seeds.

Sow True Seed Company

sowtrueseed.com

Located in Asheville, North Carolina, this small, ethical seed company offers GMO-free seeds, including many of the herbs discussed in this book.

CONVERSIONS

METRIC CONVERSION BY WEIGHT/DRY

U. S.	METRIC
¼ tsp	1 g
½ tsp	2 g
1 teaspoon	5 g
1 tablespoon	15 g
¼ ounce	7 g
½ ounce	14 g
¾ ounce	21 g
1 ounce	28 g
1/16 cup	14g
⅛ cup	28g
¼ cup	56g
⅓ cup	75g
½ cup	112g
¾ cup	168g
1 cup	224g

METRIC CONVERSION BY VOLUME/LIQUID

U. S.	METRIC
¼ teaspoon	1.25 mL
½ teaspoon	2.5 mL
1 teaspoon	5 mL
1 tablespoon	15 mL
1/16 cup	15 mL
⅛ cup	30 mL
¼ cup	60 mL
⅓ cup	80 mL
½ cup	120 mL
⅔ cup	160 mL
¾ cup	180 mL
1 cup	240 mL

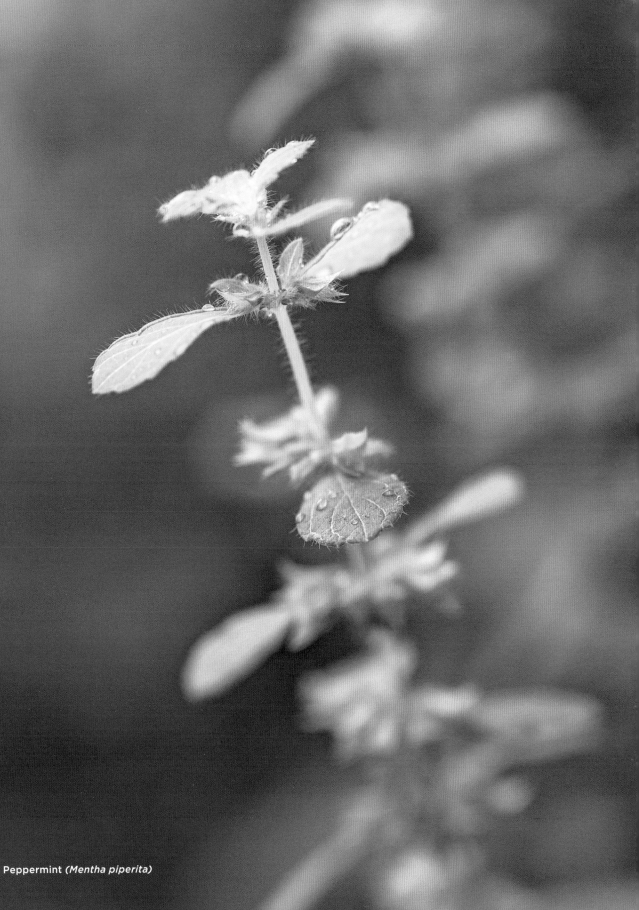

Peppermint *(Mentha piperita)*

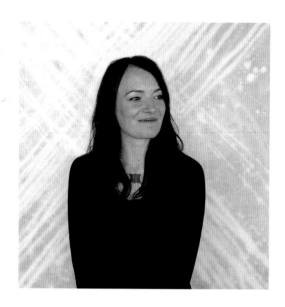

ABOUT THE AUTHOR

Heather Lee Houdek was born in Chicago, but has deep roots in Western North Carolina where she has resided most of her life. A love of plants and the natural world was instilled in her by her parents at an early age. She graduated from Brevard College in 2002 with a BA in Fine Art. She has studied herbalism both formally and informally for over 10 years. She received the bulk of her herbal education from the Appalachia School of Holistic Herbalism, where she has also taught classes. She currently works as the office manager for the American Herbalists Guild and lives in Asheville, NC, with her family of humans, animals, and plants.

ACKNOWLEDGMENTS

This lovely book would not have been possible without help from the following people: Ceara Foley and the Appalachia School of Holistic Herbalism for introducing me to many of these teachings about herbs and for her help in gathering plants; Meredith Greene for allowing me to harvest herbs out of her garden to photograph; Sandi Ford for allowing us to wander her beautiful property photographing her plants; Juniper and John O'Dell for harvesting and delivering oats to be photographed. Linda Kopp, Nicole McConville, and the wonderful folks at Lark for working with me, supporting me, and giving me the opportunity to take on this dream project.

I would also like to thank the following people: My girls – Krystie Compton-Ecks, Anne Osterman, Gwynne Rukenbrod, Kara Arndt Irani, Emily Fligg, and Davie Roberts (honorary girl)—thank you for keeping me grounded and making me laugh; Mimi Hernandez and the American Herbalists Guild, for your support, input and understanding in this endeavor; Cody Stafford, for patiently reading the rough text and your kind help, encouragement, and support with editing (and also for being an amazing roommate and brother-in-law); Michael Lance Compton for being the best boyfriend ever. I probably would not have been able to do this without your encouragement. You are the love of my life.

Most of all, I would like to thank my beautiful, talented, smart, and spectacular sisters, Sarah and Amanda. Sarah, thank you for sharing your editing, ideas, support, and creativity for this text. I am so grateful for your keen intelligence and our hours of conversation and laughter; we have lived together so long, I can't imagine not living with you! Amanda, thank you for lending your supplies, recipes, and ideas to this project. I love our shopping trips, fancy drinks, and texts and giggles. You both mean the world to me. I would not be me without you and your love.

This book is dedicated to my mother, Donna Mae Schrank Houdek. She was a DIY queen way before it was cool.

EDITOR: Linda Kopp
ART DIRECTOR & COVER DESIGNER: Kristi Pfeffer
PHOTOGRAPHER: Lynne Harty

INDEX